The Truth About Sex

A SEX PRIMER FOR THE 21ST CENTURY

Volume I: Sex and the Self

by

Dr. Gloria G. Brame

D1158769

CCB Publishing, British Columbia, Canada

The Truth About Sex, A Sex Primer for the 21st Century
Volume I: Sex and the Self

Copyright ©2011 by Dr. Gloria G. Brame
ISBN-13 978-1-926918-55-6
First Edition

Library and Archives Canada Cataloguing in Publication
Brame, Gloria G., 1955-
The truth about sex : a sex primer for the 21st century volume I : sex and
the self / by Gloria G. Brame.
ISBN 978-1-926918-55-6
Also available in electronic format.
1. Sex. I. Title.
HQ21.B7 2011   306.7   C2011-902652-X

Cover artwork and interior layout by David Ampola.

Extreme care has been taken to ensure that all information presented in
this book is accurate and up to date at the time of publishing. Neither the
author nor the publisher can be held responsible for any errors or omissions.
Additionally, neither is any liability assumed for damages resulting from the
use of the information contained herein.

Publisher: CCB Publishing
              British Columbia, Canada
              www.ccbpublishing.com

Contents

—(SECTION TWO)—

Thinking about Sex

A Note About Case Studies:
To protect the confidentiality of my clients, all case studies in this book are composites of at least two to four different patients who presented with similar problems. Names are fictitious to further protect their privacy.

YOU who celebrate bygones!
I project the history of the future.

—⁓ Walt Whitman

Section One

—⚬⚬⚬—

MASTURBATION AND ORGASM

⊰ Introduction ⊱

———◄○►———

Sex Matters

Some years ago, my mother peevishly inquired, "When are you going to write a book that won't embarrass me?" She was dismayed that her nice Jewish daughter studied a subject that she considered dirty. To her, sex was a private, embarrassing act, like using the toilet. It was disgusting to discuss it openly, much less spend time brooding over what goes on "down there." It's down there, for goodness sake.

Most of us are raised to believe that sex doesn't — or at least, shouldn't — matter. It shouldn't even matter that much in marriage. In fact, nice people shouldn't spend too much time thinking about sex. As the social narrative goes, if civilization is the sum of our intellectual achievements, then sex is the shameful burden of our primal roots. It's dirty. It's something you have to do to have children so put it off as long as possible and then just close your eyes and do it. Preferably with the lights off.

It's a strange dogma to apply to one of humanity's greatest and most enduring obsessions. Whether or not you talk about it, you cannot escape sex. Sex is all around us all the time — in the texts we send and the sites we visit, in the catcalls from construction workers on the street, in the hot outfit your neighbor's wearing, in the bouquet of flowers someone's bringing home to a sweetheart. Sex is not merely a part of life, it is integral to human life and human identity.

Human mating rituals are so seamlessly threaded throughout human life that we don't realize that many casual behaviors are in fact spurred by sexuality. You see, sex is not just all around us, it is inside of us. Sex traits are in our genes, sexual chemistry floods our brain and our bloodstream. The brain continually conveys sexual information to our entire system. The brain perceives sexual opportunity, prepares us for intimacy (or a "mating opportunity"), and when we engage in sex, our brain causes a chain reaction of events that bring us to orgasm and reward us with a flow of beneficial brain chemicals, such as oxytocin, vasopressin, serotonin and prolactin, all of which enhance mood and relaxation.

There is overwhelming evidence that sexual happiness and satisfaction promote a longer, healthier life. In a 1999 study of 3,500 adults, Dr. David Weeks, an American psychologist, was able to show that people who have sex at least three times a week look 10 years younger than their real age. Sex promotes blood circulation and cardiovascular function, improves muscle tone, and lowers the risk of stroke and heart attack. Brain chemicals released during and after orgasm contain natural opiates which combat pain, depression and stress. Sex hormones influence our moods, productivity, and social function; they profoundly impact our mental stability. Without the hormones that steer sexuality throughout out lives, the emotional experience of being human would be completely altered. Sex is at the core of human identity, not merely an appurtenance to human identity. Indeed, sex matters more than most of the things people uphold as more important than sex.

How and why we developed so many rules and taboos around sex has fascinated me since I worked on my first book, *Different Loving* (with co-authors William D. Brame and Jon Jacobs), a comprehensive study of sadomasochism, BDSM, and fetishes. I read scores of books and articles, focusing on original sources so I could build cultural frameworks and social history for each of the types of BDSM we covered. It became increasingly apparent that even authoritative texts on sex and sexual normalcy were profoundly flawed. Virtually all of the great 19th century theorists, for example, misunderstood, mischaracterized and discounted female sexual drive. Case studies of the day were analyzed through a filter of elitism, religious doctrine and, sometimes, sheer quackery. Nor did the situation measurably improve in the medico-forensic establishment throughout the 20th century, as psychiatrists and courts continued to rely heavily on the biased opinions rendered in the 19th century. While new discoveries have changed the face of virtually all the social sciences, and public attitudes towards sex had undergone numerous revolutionary changes, underlying attitudes about sex itself were literally frozen in Victorian time.

By the time I was working on my next volume on kinky sex (*Come Hither: A Commonsense Guide to Kinky Sex*), I was obsessed with this problem. I was in the last stages of completing my Ph.D. in human sexuality, and like every grad student, had a mania for reading and collecting data. I read, for example, the sobering statistics that 31% of all men and 43% of all women in the U.S. are sexually dysfunctional (*Journal of the American Medical Association*, 1999). The following year, *American Family Physician* reported that over 50% of women were dysfunctional because they cannot achieve orgasm from intercourse and 15% have never had an orgasm at all. I started adding up the numbers. The National Institute of Health estimates that 30 million American men are impotent and tens of millions more have problems with low libido, premature ejaculation, and orgasm disorders. 15% of men and 30% of women have Hypoactive Sex Disorder, (*Endocrinology Review*, 2001), the clinical term for lack of desire. Dysfunction everywhere one turns, or so it would seem.

It struck me then that, perhaps, the problem was not that Americans were spiraling into mass dysfunction but rather that the interpretations of the data were fruit from the poison tree. If our model of what is normal is flawed, our definition of things like "dysfunction" and "perversion" must be flawed too. Did the medical researchers ask all these dysfunctional people if they thought they could be more orgasmic from a different type of sex? Were some of the subjects secretly gay or lesbian and thus would never find complete sexual fulfillment from heterosexual acts?

What if some cases of dysfunction are in fact the product of people continually trying to have a type of sex that doesn't actually turn them on because they believe that is the only type of sex they are allowed to have? If 50% of women can't orgasm from vaginal intercourse, instead of calling that a dysfunction, perhaps — as most sexologists today would agree — vaginal intercourse isn't quite as sexually important to all female sexual function as commonly assumed. Today's therapist would encourage such women to experiment with vibrators, fingers, tongues and sexual fantasies. If they can enjoy the experience and achieve climax, it is not a true dysfunction.

When everyone is held to the same pre-emptive model of how they are *supposed* to feel sexually, it's inevitable that a sizeable segment of the population will always be dysfunctional or considered perverts or weirdos. As things stand, we live in an age when most people still hold their great-grandparents' belief that masturbation is bad or wrong, while data are released weekly showing that orgasms are vital to human health. There is a cognitive dissonance between the facts about sex and the beliefs about sex. Missionary-position sex is still believed to be the "best" or "most natural" type of sex even though a 2010 study by the Kinsey Institute demonstrated that oral sex is actually the most popular type of sex.

The schisms in our culture's attitudes towards sex are cracking wide open, in part because of Internet culture. In 2006, *Babytalk* magazine created a furor when an issue's cover showed a woman breast feeding a baby; although no nipple was visible, 25% of readers protested that the image was pornographic. A few months later, the infamous "2 girls, 1 cup," a trailer for a hard core copraphilia video, became an Internet sensation. It is not, as some prudes might have it, that depravity is taking over; it's that sexual beliefs about what is and is not permissible, or what is and isn't normal, do not mirror actual human sexual behavior. Real human sexuality is, and always has been, diverse.

When I set up my private practice in 2000, my clients' needs for better information about sex pushed me to examine new and more urgent questions about the role of sex in daily existence. I had expected to see depression and despair in victims of abuse, but I had never appreciated how unhappy life felt for people who experience sex as a stressful or distasteful act. Whether it was the woman who had never had an orgasm with her husband, or the man who said that intercourse was nothing more to him than masturbating into a sleeve, people felt incomplete, and somehow inferior to those who they imagined were having hot, passionate sex — which they, naturally, believed was everyone in the world but themselves.

Sex matters. My clients convince me of that every day. Each problem, each life story, continually shapes and reshapes my perspectives on sex as it is truly lived, and gives me new tools to unlock its mysteries. This book encompasses the cumulative knowledge I've applied to my practice, set out for the first time in writing. Using social histories of sex, and relying on hundreds of sex studies, my mission here is to build evidence-based models of human sexuality. I also use composite case studies (to protect the identities of my clients) to give the dry facts a warm human face and to show how sex truly and deeply impacts people's lives, relationships, self-image, and mental health.

Why We Don't Know What We Know about Sex

Imagine if our current understanding and treatment of diseases were based on what people believed 130 years ago. Barbers would perform surgeries, blood-letters would leech us, caustic enemas and emetics would be daily rituals, and the bumps on our head might figure in our treatment plan. We have come an astonishing distance from the magical thinking, charlatanism, alchemy, and fraud that dominated medicine until the 20th century.

Yet, our ideas about sex remain welded to antiquated beliefs first articulated by ancient Greco-Roman philosophers. Echoing Aristotelian theory, Roman philosophers posited that sexual desire poisoned the mind with passions and drained men of virility. Seneca boiled it down to a simple edict: "Do nothing for the sake of pleasure." The philosopher Artemidorus declared that missionary position intercourse was the only moral form of sex and pronounced oral sex an abomination.

The Greco-Roman concepts of sex for pleasure as a morally weakening force received perhaps its most critical advocacy a millennium later in the work of Saint Thomas of Aquinas, whose opinions became the basis of European and American beliefs about sex for the next five centuries. In essence, Aquinas retrofitted the sexual theories of the pagans to Roman Catholic purposes. Aquinas asserted that sex served only one purpose in life: reproduction. Bearing children was a sacred duty. Sex merely for pleasure was a sin, even when the partners were married.

It was only in the 19th century that belief-based ideologies began, at last, to shift in favor of the growing evidence that sex was a truly complex phenomenon. With the blossoming of medicine in the mid 19th century, some of the greatest minds of the Victorian age — most notably Sigmund Freud — set about unraveling the meaning and biology of sex. For the first time, sexual behaviors were classified, categorized, diagnosed and treated by medical doctors.

Unfortunately, by modern standards, Victorian science was woefully unscientific. While the doctors themselves were serious men, some of their conclusions were absurd. The fatal flaw in Victorian sexology was that, in their eagerness to establish diagnostic models of sexuality, they never asked the single most important question: "What is normal sexuality?" Instead, they assumed they already knew what it was: vaginal sex in marriage for the purpose of reproduction. (I'll call it the Reproductive Model and will use RM as short-hand from here on.)

While they analyzed hundreds, perhaps thousands, of cases which contradicted their assumptions, rather than question the validity of those assumptions as a good scientist should, they diagnosed everyone who did not conform to their expectations as being mentally unbalanced and in need of psychiatric intervention. They assumed that women by nature do not have independent sex drives. They believed that masturbation caused debilitating disease. For decades after, women with high sex-drives, masturbators, hedonists, homosexuals, transpeople and others who defied the Victorian standard were subject to involuntary treatments and hospitalizations.

Today, we have an exuberance of data across numerous medical specialties that prove just how wrong our predecessors were to limit their definition of normalcy to reproductive function.

Diversity is Normal

Think of all the people you know who have had casual sex, one-night stands, same-sex encounters, or threesomes. Add to that all the people who watch adult movies, surf porn, sext, go to strip clubs, patronize call-girls, and get happy endings at massage parlors. Then think of the tens of millions of North Americans who identify as swingers, bisexuals, gay, kinky, polyamorous or fetishist, and the scores of millions who enjoy sexual role-play, fantasies, new positions, and sensual adult toys. By Victorian standards, all of the above are deviants. Yet if you eliminate all of the above populations, just how many "normal" adults are left?

After 20+ years of sexual research and 11 in clinical practice, I have come to realize that it's only the tiniest minority of people who faithfully adhere to the RM by choice. Even the most conservative and religious people will grant themselves some leeway when it comes to sex. Cosmo magazine makes it sound new every time, but oral sex techniques were undoubtedly old news to adults long before Ancient Rome was founded.

Perhaps most telling of all are the lessons of history. No matter how many repressive regimes have come and gone, no matter how many laws and religious mandates dictate sexual behaviors, no matter how much persecution a sexual minority may endure, each new generation repeats the sexual patterns of preceding ones. This suggests a biological basis that surpasses cultural expectations. It is reasonable to conclude that the reason adults may find it difficult to conform to the traditional standard is because the social standard conflicts with their biological make-up.

I see the individual suffering that confusion about sex and normalcy causes people. I also see that knowledge, education and the simple truths about sex, delivered candidly without judgment, alleviates that pain. Throwing out some of the old beliefs about how sex "should be" and embracing the evidence about how sex is actually lived is profoundly therapeutic.

A Universal Solution

To move forward, we can't keep pretending that sex is a less vital concern to the quality of human life than history or philosophy or literature. Sex is one of humanity's central obsessions. Whether we're browsing porn or signing petitions to stop porn, whether we're taking tantric courses to expand our orgasmic potential or trying to pray away our lust, whether our sex lives are an oasis of joy or a pit of torment, we are all preoccupied with sex.

Sex is with us from birth to death. Sexual events occur undetected inside your body, as our hormones fluctuate according to moods, life events and aging. Sexual emotions are happening in your home, whether you are celibate or sexually active. Sexual events occur in our private worlds — whether it's an affair at the office, a scandal at one's place of worship, or a sex club moving into one's neighborhood.

The time is overdue for a modern dialogue about sex and new models of normalcy based on the facts we know instead of the beliefs our ancestors held in the absence of knowledge.

⊰ Chapter One ⊱

Masturbation

————◄o►————

The Trouble with Masturbation

The most fundamental sexual behavior known to humans has been shrouded by so many myths and dogma over time that most adults have no idea what's normal. Even people who are reasonably open-minded about the topic still suspect that, at heart, masturbation is dangerous or unhealthy, particularly if you "do it too much."

"Too much" is not an objective standard. There is no such thing as "too much sex" if the person having that sex is enjoying it, remains healthy, and continues to derive pleasure from other aspects of life (career, family, spirituality, etc.). Equally important, what is too much for one person isn't enough for another. Yet I've spoken to hundreds of men and women over the years who believed that something was wrong with them simply because they liked to masturbate.

Rodger M. walked into my office, head down, jaw set. A tall serious man in his 20s, he glanced around nervously, as if checking for hidden cameras, then sank into a chair. I wondered what grim tale he would reveal — was he a rapist? A convicted child molester? I began asking basic questions while he shifted and avoided my eyes.

He interrupted me, "Look Doc. Here's the problem. I jerk off too much. I'm an addict."

Rodger had visited a website where he took an "Are you a sex addict?" quiz prepared by someone who bills himself as the pre-eminent expert in sex addiction, and with every answer, Rodger sank into deeper gloom. Yes, he looked at porn. Yes, he jerked off. He even looked at porn while he jerked off. According to the site, Rodger was a sex addict.

"Really?" I asked. I ran through a series of basic questions: Was he functioning at work? Did he have a decent social life? Stable relationships? Stable finances? Did masturbation interfere with any of those? Was anyone being hurt by his behavior? At the end I said, "You're doing great at work, you have an active social life, and you make good choices. I don't think you're an addict."

"So why do I jerk off so much?"

"Perhaps you like it," I smiled. "I know I do."

He blushed. "Yeah, yeah, I do. At least until I start worrying about it."

This, of course, is the biggest problem with masturbation; not the masturbation itself, which is without doubt the single most ubiquitous, universal behavior, but the guilt, the shame, the anxiety, even the despair that people suffer over it.

I asked him how often he masturbated for it to cause him enough concern to visit a sex therapist. Rodger told me once or twice a day. I told him that I recommend that male clients have a sexual release once a day for health reasons, he laughed in surprise.

"Medical studies have proven that men who masturbate five times a week reduce their risk of prostate cancer by up to 60%. You can confirm that with your urologist," I said. "Orgasm plays a vital role in male sexual health. So I think you're in good shape. In fact, I'd be concerned if you only masturbated a few times a month. Daily orgasms are one of the best things you can do for yourself."

Rodger told me that since his teens he had been tormented with anxiety because he was told that jerking off was wrong. He worried that if he did it every day, he'd turn into a "pathetic freak" or that he wouldn't be able to get it up anymore. I gently let him know that his constant worrying and guilt trips were more likely to damage his health than masturbation.

I take a holistic approach in therapy. I believe that sex always spills into daily life and vice versa; if Rodger was shirking responsibilities or fleeing intimacy to escape into masturbation, I would consider it problematic. Simply to enjoy yourself with something that harms no one (including yourself) is not a problem.

I continued asking him questions about his life and habits. Other than his anxieties about masturbation he was fairly happy, upbeat, and high-functioning. Looking at the whole of Rodger's life, it was also obvious that he had much more control over his impulses than he'd credited himself for having. We talked about his personal history and background. He was raised in a conservative household where sex was never discussed. When the subject arose, the message from his parents was clear: sex was dirty, undignified, taboo. The only acceptable sex occurred between husband and wife. In Rodger's mind, by masturbating he was, in effect, disappointing his family and at risk of disgrace should anyone ever find out.

I gave him all the latest and greatest information culled from studies on the voluminous benefits of masturbation. When I informed him that having an orgasm daily is physically healthier than not having one, he was at first stunned, then palpably relieved.

The man who came to my office afraid that his daily masturbation meant he was an addict was transformed by that conversation. It alleviated a burden of shame he had carried since he was twelve. More often than not, clients like Rodger don't need to see a sex therapist more than once or twice. Sometimes, once they finally admit what they always considered a "terrible secret," they already feel better and more in control. Putting voice to their fears and then realizing that they are just fears, not realities, is in itself deeply therapeutic.

What Is Masturbation?

Masturbation is the fundamental building block of adult sexual performance. It is the first step we take towards defining what we like sexually and learning how our bodies respond to sexual stimulation. Consciously, we may be driven by nothing more than the fact that it feels good but, developmentally, masturbation teaches us how to elicit and control our sexual responses and, most importantly, to achieve the all-important sexual release.

Margo L. was a 50-something woman, married to Jim, her high school sweetheart. They had several children but Margo had never had an orgasm with Jim and now, facing menopause, was frightened she never would. She was angry and blamed Jim for being cold and selfish. Jim wanted sex almost every night, had his orgasm, and turned over to go to sleep, leaving her awake and frustrated. He didn't seem to care how she felt. Early on, he tried harder and did some foreplay, she said, but he'd long since given up and only focused on his own needs. She was hurt to the point of rage about Jim's attitudes. He made her feel unloved and unappreciated. She had packed her bags more than once. Sex was all about him and she just didn't want to do it anymore. Having sex with Jim only served as a grim reminder of how empty it made her feel. At the same time, she really didn't want a divorce — he was a good husband and great father — so she continued to engage in sex that she found joyless.

In the course of taking her sexual history, I asked her at what age she had started masturbating. There was a long pause. She never masturbated. She was raised in a different time, she said, a time when women didn't do that sort of thing. So it wasn't just that she didn't have orgasms with her husband. She said she'd never had an orgasm at all. She was raised to believe that sex was reserved for marriage, and so she waited to be married, with the expectation that once they began having sex, she would learn to enjoy it. Instead, she had been waiting all those years for Jim to figure out what would work and then do it to her. As she saw it, her sexual pleasure was entirely in his hands — and he had failed her as a husband by refusing to provide it.

She was first hostile, then humbled, when I told her that if you don't know how to give yourself an orgasm, chances of someone else knowing how to do it are slim to nil. Two sexually healthy adults can have orgasms together if both of them want the experience and each of them knows what it takes to achieve that climax. Exactly how they get there varies enormously but the better you know how to achieve your own orgasm, the greater your chances of having one with someone else. There are always marvelous exceptions — the magical lover who seems to know exactly how to touch you and where and in what way and at what moment. Sadly, such serendipitous occasions are rare. Infinitely more common are adults who suffer for years because they don't know how to give themselves orgasms or how to be orgasmic with partners.

Margo's belief that her orgasm was entirely up to her husband virtually guaranteed that she would never climax. She didn't understand her own sexual anatomy or response. She assumed that because she couldn't climax from five minutes of thrusting after perfunctory, almost non-existent foreplay, something was wrong with her. She should have known better; she'd read enough on the subject to understand the importance of foreplay for women. But she was so hurt and embarrassed by what she viewed as her own inadequacy, that she didn't know how to ask for more and immediately backed down when her husband didn't show an interest in giving her more.

Margo's problems were deeper than orgasmic capability, beginning with her passivity and low self-esteem. In addition to talking through all her deeper issues, I gave her assignments to begin the process of learning how to give herself pleasure, including gentle exploration of her genitals in the shower, and the purchase of a simple vibrator. A few months into therapy, Margo excitedly reported that she had finally achieved the orgasm which had eluded her for 50 years. She now understood that the key for her was a long slow build-up, with a lot of caressing and kissing to tease her into readiness. I could see the positive changes in her mood, body, language, and eyes. Margo looked as happy as a kid with a new toy.

How Do People Masturbate?

While the act of masturbation is universal — most sexually healthy people engage in it — there are numerous variables that account for differences in the hows, whys, and wherefores of solo sex. Not all masturbation leads to orgasm. In people with orgasmic dysfunctions or organic health issues, orgasm may be elusive or weak. Some forms of masturbation are focused on the feelings of arousal and excitement: orgasm may be deferred for another time.

The range of ways adults may experience arousal and satisfaction from solo sex are ultimately an aggregate of biology, environment, and opportunity. Even when two people use the same exact techniques in masturbating, one should assume that they still don't "feel" it the same way. Some people become giddily overwhelmed by pleasurable sensations to their erotic spots, and others maintain a relaxed, somewhat unchanged affect during the act. Typical or normal responses are somewhere in the middle range: a feeling of anticipation and excitement, coupled with deep pleasure, completed with a powerful experience of relief.

Masturbation in men typically means manual stimulation of the penis, usually rubbing it up and down. In women, it typically involves manual stimulation of the clitoris or pressure applied to the genital region. It's also typical for adults to enhance the sensuality of masturbation using vibrators, dildos, jack-off devices, bondage toys, lotions, lubes, and a range of other genital-centric appliances and stimulants.

Commonly, people give themselves sensations in other parts of their bodies before and during masturbation. Garden-variety adjuncts include self-stimulation of vagina, nipples and anus, often using sex toys such as dildos, butt plugs, vibrators, or anal probes. Probably even more common are the "sex toys of opportunity," or random objects that you adapt to sexual purposes. When I was 15, I "borrowed" a friend's electric shaver for a quick orgasmic romp before cleaning it and returning it to her drawer. I felt ashamed of myself, but not so ashamed that I didn't continue to have casual sex with common objects in my parents' home throughout my randy teens, always tidying up the crime scenes so no one ever found out.

Sexual self-experiments are entirely normal. They go along with our innate curiosity about our bodies' reactions to stimulants and our inborn cravings for variety. It's typical for us to experiment with soft sensations, such as the way rose petals or silks feel on our skin. It's also typical to experiment with intense sensations, such as pinching or slapping ourselves during masturbation. All such experiments are natural impulses to explore the boundaries of our innate sensuality, and determine which sets of sensations give us the most pleasure. Individual biology accounts for what places will feel best, while hormones, aging, emotional issues, and physical illness all alter sensitivity and sexual responsiveness throughout our lives.

Carl P. started masturbating when he was about fourteen, and engaged in the typical stroking behavior. But even at that young age, he didn't find the stroking to be enough sensation for him. His masturbation always involved some other sensual element: either he handled his penis roughly, or pinched his own nipples, or he attached clothespins to his scrotum or all of the above. As enjoyable as he found the stroking, he needed the additional stimuli to climax. Some might call Carl a sensation junkie; others might call him a masochist. As a sexologist, I just consider Carl to be a guy who has a high natural drive for intense sensation. When I asked Carl about his other interests I learned he was passionate about extreme sports. He was also the guy who ordered the spiciest dish on the menu when he went out with friends. He proudly admitted he'd won a few "bet that's too hot for you to eat" wagers in his time. I wasn't surprised to discover that his social identity mirrored his sexual identity.

From a sexological point of view, the sexually healthiest person is the one who enjoys exploring his or her full potential for pleasure. Culturally, we poke fun at masturbation and mock those who invest in a lot of sex toys or, worse, question their character, as if the pursuit of sexual ecstasy is, in itself, morally degrading.

To a sexologist, it's the opposite: the most sexually balanced people are the ones who are least confined by assumptions and expectations about what they "should" like and, instead, take the organic approach by simply testing themselves to see what they actually do like. I've occasionally remarked that the most perverse type of sexuality is when someone believes they have to perform a particular act that turns them off again, or when they settle on one method of giving or receiving pleasure and never again vary from it.

People who masturbate in only one specific way for their entire lives — never varying the routine, never discovering whether another spot on his or her body could be a source of sensuality — miss out on the greatest part of sexuality: the delight of variety. If you think about every other area of human life — music, food, beverages — variety is the rule. How often do you find yourself at a stranger's house and discover they use your favorite brands of shampoo, toothpaste and soap? To believe in one monolithic model of how, when and how often to masturbate is as irrational as believing everyone is morally obligated to use Crest toothpaste on their teeth and Ivory soap in the shower.

Indeed, the person far most likely to develop problems with masturbation is the one who (a) does it the least and (b) does it the same exact way every time. Some adults have to retrain themselves when their masturbatory pattern has been so fixed for so long that they cannot get the kind of sensation they need from penetrative or other types of partnered sex. If you spend twenty years of your life only succeeding in climaxing from one single method of masturbation, your likelihood of making an easy shift to a partner-based sex life may be challenging because unless your partner can reproduce that exact same sensation, you may find it hard to come.

In nature — without inhibitions, taboos, traumas, and the collective weight of civilization — there is no doubt that nearly all human beings would experiment with every possible variety of self-pleasure. We want to feel good. We love things that taste good, smell good, look good, sound good, and feel good. If we were not raised to separate our pelvic region from the rest of our bodies, we would explore liberally, front and back, until we found exactly the right set of sensations that brought us the greatest level of sexual satisfaction. But we do not live in nature, so it is the rare individual who feels empowered to strive for enhanced sexual pleasure.

While circumstances can alter or deform the natural development of masturbatory instincts, the good news is that behaviors you learn can be unlearned. However, retraining yourself to orgasm from different stimuli requires a serious commitment to behavior modification. As I frequently remind clients, if you keep doing the same things, you're going to get the same results. There are no absolute guarantees that behavioral modification will work, but I've yet to see a truly motivated client fail to make positive changes in his or her sex life.

Frank Z., a handsome man in his late 30s, grew up in a large family with virtually no privacy. As a teen, he developed a furtive method of masturbation, stroking quickly, trying to bring himself to climax as fast as he could. He became expert at sliding his hand into his pants to rub himself off discreetly and tested himself a few times as a teen by doing so in public places, unnoticed. He'd long since given up the habit of public masturbation but still had a taste for fast sex — something which his lovers routinely complained about. Frank was a pragmatic, stoic guy: to him, orgasm was the only goal of sex. Privately, he sneered at "too much fooling around," which he viewed as somewhat effeminate. He believed every man just wanted to get their rocks off with the least amount of bother and fuss.

In order for Frank to achieve a healthier, and more mutually satis-fying sex life, he was going to have to slow down and learn to enjoy the journey. The challenge was to move him off his life-long habit of goal-oriented sex and focus on pleasure-oriented sex. Since he was neither shy nor inhibited about his body, I suggested that he relearn its possibilities by exploring sensations in every area except his penis. I told him to start with his toes and work his way up, inch by inch, front and back. He could do it with a partner or solo, in bed or in a relaxing bath. I encouraged him to give him-self challenges: other than his penis, what was the most sensitive spot on his body? Although he found the exercises frustrating and even annoying at the beginning, he agreed to abstain from direct stimulation to his genitals for a week. During that time, his job was to figure out what other types of stimulation aroused him and whether any other sensations could bring him to climax. Since Frank worked in a hospital and was all too familiar with patients who were unable to give themselves direct stimulation, I suggest-ed he imagine what it would be like if he was in their position: how would he go about deriving sexual pleasure if he could not quickly, effectively masturbate with his hand?

By refreshing his palette and directing him away from instant gratification, Frank discovered a world of new sensation he had not previously considered. It took only a few weeks before he was eager to explore these new understandings of his body with his lover, Don, who was stunned when Frank offered to turn the tables, and see which spots made him extra happy as well. Of course, there were still times when Frank liked to get off in a hurry but the better he became in bed, the more patient he grew and the more willing he was to let orgasm take a backseat to sensuality. When Don told him he had turned into a wonderfully versatile and skilled lover, Frank felt like a completely new, and much happier, man.

Another patient, John R., a newlywed in his mid 20s, was having difficulty adjusting to married sex because he kept expecting to feel all the same things he felt during masturbation when he made love to his wife, Kendra. Since boyhood, John had masturbated in one specific way and had inadvertently conditioned himself to climax from that one method — which involved a lot of tugging and rough sensation to his penis. After only six months of marriage, he was already locking himself in the bathroom to relieve his sexual tension. Although he was very attracted to Kendra, he was too embarrassed to admit what he liked and couldn't bring himself to tell his beloved that their sex life didn't satisfy him. Happily for him, Kendra was willing and eager to make changes and, at my recommendation, came with him to his next session. I recommended that they start out by simply exploring mutual masturbation — with him coaching her on the sensations he liked the most. Kendra wasn't just a loving woman, she was a smart one with a strong dominant streak. She took to rough play like a duck to water, and quickly figured out the kinds of sensations that sent him through the roof. They were both shocked to realize how intense their chemistry could be once they gave themselves permission to reveal ALL their secrets. The more he told his wife about his hot buttons and fantasies, the more she confessed her own. In just two months, they began a truly adult, mature, loving model of sex, based on what made them happiest.

A meaningful consideration in figuring out what you, personally, need from sex is that innumerable physical variables make one person's sexual response different from another's. Human genitals are as different in their minutiae as hands or feet. Size and color are the most apparent differences but subtle variations, internal and external, are the rule. Not all genitals are positioned exactly the same: your parts may be slightly higher or lower, further up front or further back, than the next person's. The distance between genitals and anus vary. Some of your genital aspects may be more prominent or less prominent. You may have hair where someone else is (naturally) bare. You may have a curve where someone else is straight, or wrinkles where the next person is smooth. Your veins may be closer to the surface, and your nerves may cluster in slightly higher concentrations. Your overall skin sensitivity may be low, medium or high. Such normal physical variations contribute to differences in sensitivity and response; the same caress or stroke that feels fantastic to one person could feel painful to another and won't feel like anything at all to a third.

Lena R. was a vibrant, optimistic woman in her late 20s. She had freely explored her body and her sensuality since childhood. Her favorite activity was pulling the bed-sheets tight between her legs and riding them until "the oooh feeling," as she described it.

Sometimes she added other things — a shampoo bottle, a bar of soap — to increase the intensity of the pressure against her vulva. In her college years, she'd sown all her wild oats and then some, but one thing still eluded her: being able to climax during intercourse. Now in a happy marriage, she still couldn't orgasm unless something was pressed tight against her labia over the clitoral hood. As we talked, it struck me that Lena wasn't "stuck" on any one type of masturbatory habit. She had experimented with dozens of different ways of reaching climax. But in every case, the method that put her over the top invariably involved pressure on the outside of the vulva. She volunteered that once, by accident, her husband pressed down hard on her pelvis during sex and she "almost" came. She was frustrated by her lifelong inability to climax from penetration and wondered if she'd "masturbated too much" as a girl and ruined her chances of being able to enjoy "normal" sex.

Contrary to the popular image of women masturbating in ways that mimic the pleasures of intercourse — an image belabored in pornography for men — in my clinical experience, female orgasm commonly derives from pressure, friction, and other sensation either to the outside or visible aspects of female genitals (such as the clitoris, labia, and pubic mound). Vaginal penetration is wildly exciting to some women, but for many others, it is primarily an adjunct to their pleasures (or fantasies), not the mechanism for their orgasm. This is, indeed, one of the reasons why foreplay is so important. Stroking, caressing and other manipulations to female genitalia prepare a woman for orgasm.

Getting to understand your individual anatomy is a vital piece of the puzzle in successful masturbation and climax. Endocrinologists use a term I love: genital congestion. It may sound as if you have a cold in your groin but it's the opposite: it's a measure of blood-flow (and subsequent warmth), based on the amount of swelling that occurs. Depending on your sexual health, genetic traits, and vascular fitness, swelling in the genitals (penis, clitoris, vagina, and testicles) can range from truly impressive to barely noticeable. Some men find that their penis in repose is small but that they grow surprisingly large when fully erect; others may seem well-endowed, but do not see significant lengthening during erection; and most men fall between the two ends of the spectrum. Similar variations are common in women in as well. Some are endowed with a clitoris that swells significantly and protrudes from the labia; others show little or limited clitoral growth during arousal.

Some people experience genital congestion as a light, tingling pleasure; some as a swooningly sharp pang; some as a desperate clawing need for relief. All of these little (or not so little) variations impinge on what kind of pressure you need on your genitals as well.

Many of the women I've worked with admit that they still masturbate as they did as little girls, only in place of blankets or objects, they now use vibrators. Indeed, one of the most popular vibrators ever sold — the "Magic Wand," manufactured by Hitachi — is a non-penetrative toy. As sex toys for women become more sophisticated, the emphasis has trended away from penetrative toys. The most upscale new tinglers focus on stimulating the clitoris and external genital region. Abundant anecdotal material proves again and again that, in private, for many different reasons, women opt for non-penetrative masturbation. Wishing you were built slightly differently, or could climax from things that biologically don't work for you, is, in my opinion, a recipe for dysfunction. Far better for every woman to accept that her body is unique, to map its sweetest spots, and then to exploit her natural sensuality.

I suggested to Lena that instead of reaching for a goal that may never be possible, we assume it was natural for her to need pressure to climax. It was entirely possible that the location of her clit, or the sensitive nerves concentrated behind the clit, meant that her body simply responded best when stimulation was applied from the outside, not the inside. If this was how she was anatomically geared, she could fight and ultimately lose, or work with her body to find new pathways to coupled orgasm. We reviewed different sex positions and movements that could increase pressure on her pelvic region — from having him manually apply pressure during sex (placing his hand over her mound and pushing down), to doggie-style sex with something under her pelvis that she could grind against. Knowing they were very creative and open-minded, I requested that she allow him to watch her masturbate so he could better understand what she did to climax. It might give him ideas about what he could add to the mix. They agreed to try a range of new techniques and were thrilled with the results. They found one sure-fire method that worked for them — he entered her from behind and clamped his hand over her genitals, squeezing and rubbing as he moved in and out of her. It worked so well they had their first-ever simultaneous orgasm.

The last variable in how people masturbate depends on how much time and effort they invest in learning their own bodies' responses and how good they get at giving themselves pleasure. In the pursuit of more intensely arousing masturbation, males have been known to penetrate an impressive range of bizarre objects. My personal favorite was in the novel *Portnoy's Complaint* where the eponymous protagonist masturbated in a hunk of raw meat slated to be cooked for dinner that night. Gross, perhaps, but honest. Virtually anything which can be penetrated has been penetrated by men in search of satisfaction.

Women are also known to be curiously incautious in their choices of inanimate partners. I once advised some lawyers who were trying to analyze the legality of images appearing on their site. We all gained an education in the possibilities for creative excess some people bring to solo sex. I will never forget the lady who made an art of inserting wooden chair legs into her vagina. I was seriously concerned about splinters.

Insertions are a fairly common act during masturbation as an adjunct to pleasure. In addition to the most common practice (using a specialized sex toy in the vagina or the anus), people find unusual applications for other things. Some people enjoy inserting catheters and other narrow items into the urethra. Emergency room doctors have removed everything from bottles and light bulbs to baked potatoes from colons. As radical or unusual as these masturbatory games may seem to some people, in fact, doctors and helping professionals are well aware that they occur throughout the mainstream population.

As a sex therapist, I have learned that just when you think you've heard it all, you discover that of course you haven't. There are always new angles, new variations and new fantasies that make one person's masturbation different from the next. For me, frankly, that is the joy of being a sex therapist in the first place. The diversity of human sexuality is a beautiful and spiritual spectacle to behold.

Why Do People Masturbate?

As will become increasingly, almost tediously, evident as you read this book, the honest simple answer to every question regarding "Why do people do X sex act?" is the remarkably dull response, "Because it feels right to them." It feels right and it feels very good too.

I realize most of you are thinking you didn't need me to tell you masturbation feels good but it is on the notion of "right" versus "wrong" that people go astray. People who believe that sex in general is dirty are always the first to say that an act like masturbation is "wrong." They'll use expressions like "it's not healthy" or "it's a selfish pleasure" or send other messages that something so biologically natural is physically, morally or spiritually degrading. And, since masturbation is the first sexual act most humans know, we usually learn very early in life that we shouldn't do it. In truth, nothing could be more right or more natural. Our minds crave the chemicals that sex produces; our biology benefits by the catharsis of orgasm. Our bodies don't care what makes us climax as long as we do. Moreover, manually stimulating your genitals is by far the single safest kind of sex available to humans.

Humans are hardly alone in the enjoyment of solo sex. Innumerable species, including primates and house pets, engage in self-stimulation for fun. We once had a bachelor Bichon Frise with a disturbing passion for sofa pillows. Being a sex therapist, I wanted to be clinically cool about it but I couldn't help cringing when he humped the pillows like a coked-up hustler getting paid by the stroke. We ultimately broke his habit, though I admit I felt like a party-pooper for ending his happy time.

From my clinical point of view, we are hard-wired to masturbate. We don't have a choice about the impulse. It comes with the human territory. Considering how much effort has historically been expended on trying to force people to stop masturbating, if we could stop or control it we would have by now. Nor does anyone teach kids how to masturbate; if anything, they are discouraged from it, even punished for it. Yet nothing can stop the human drive to explore self-pleasure.

How Often Do People Masturbate?

As much as people lie, fudge and fib about sex, when it comes to masturbation, they lie even more. Indeed, sometimes they kid themselves and don't realize (or accept) that they are masturbating. So it is almost impossible to know for sure what people are actually doing in the privacy of their bedrooms.

When I ran a blind poll on my blog a few years ago, 75% of the 235 respondents (male and female) said they masturbated at least once a day. That number isn't scientific, but based on clinical and anecdotal experience, I think once every day is a reasonable estimate for healthy adults. Commonly, adults do it at night, as a relaxing pre-sleep ritual. (The second most common time to do it is upon waking up — for some people, a morning orgasm gives a lift to the day.) Some people benefit from masturbating two or three times a day, others will never want more than two or three orgasms a week or month. It's all normal.

That said, the number of times any given individual feels the urge to masturbate is influenced by a range of factors: opportunity, health, psychological state, even DNA may play a role. We already know that some of us are born with more vigorous libidos than others, and that some of us have higher levels of hormones than others. We also have early research demonstrating that sexual behaviors are inherited (for example, genetic testing has shown that premature ejaculation appears to be a paternal trait). But biology is not entirely destiny when it comes to sex. Environment and opportunity play mitigating roles in how often a person masturbates. Most importantly, your attitude about your genitals influences your comfort-level and the pleasure received from touching yourself.

Ed M. was a genuinely likeable, earnest, kind man in his early 30s. The only child of a religious single mother, Ed learned right from wrong early and in very black and white terms. He worshiped his mother as much as he feared her. At age 13, when Ed's mother caught him masturbating, his world came crashing in. He told me he could feel her disgust and disappointment in the core of his own soul. From then on, he vowed he would never masturbate again. He and his mother prayed for him to develop the strength to resist his urges, although he confided that, on the inside, he really didn't think he'd been doing anything wrong. He just wanted to "do the right thing" and he believed his mother knew what God expected of him.

Ever since leaving home, his old urges returned, seemingly twice as intensely. His old resolutions faded and he resumed masturbating. However, he never got over the shame and guilt of his youth. He had internalized his mother's disapproval so deeply that he literally felt he should be punished every time he touched himself. He came to me hoping I would be able to "cure" his need to masturbate. He blamed masturbation for his inability to form successful relationships with women. He was dying to get married, have children, and lead a normal life. He was convinced that his interest in masturbation was an obstacle to all that.

Ed spent a couple of years working with me on what I quickly perceived to be the genuine issue behind his angst: as much as he loved his mother, she had been such a powerful and controlling influence in his life that he was actually afraid of women; afraid of their control and afraid that they would disapprove of him as much as his mother had. His natural impulse to give himself pleasure had become confused with this fear, so that each time he masturbated he saw himself slipping further away from any possibility of marriage; yet, the more he saw himself slipping away, the more he seemed to need to masturbate. Slowly it became clear to him that his masturbation was not the problem. The real problem was his profound guilt and his mixed feelings about allowing himself to feel vulnerable around a woman. The anxiety he felt over his "weakness" merely filled him with so much tension that the only way to relieve his mind was by masturbating which, of course, only made him feel worse, and more stressed out. The vicious cycle had consumed his life.

As Ed's self-esteem improved in therapy, and as he sorted out his mother's anti-sex attitudes from his own fairly open-minded attitudes, he developed the confidence to date more. He was amazed and grateful when one woman he began seeing told him that she loved giving hand-jobs, and encouraged him to explore creative sex with her. I can't say that all of his emotional baggage from life with his mom vanished, but Ed's contentment and optimism rose spectacularly, thanks to a good sex life with an understanding and caring girlfriend, and he stopped demonizing masturbation.

Considering that they are so often punished for it, sometimes by their mothers, wives or girlfriends, sometimes by clergy, sometimes by culture itself, it's not surprising that many men struggle with emotional pain over masturbating. The culture accepts that men are highly sexed and jokes about masturbation are now as prevalent as condemnations and shaming about it. But if male masturbation gets the lion's share of public attention, it's because there is still an underlying belief in our culture that women aren't fully sexual and therefore don't need to masturbate. But we are and we do. Women just don't seem to belabor their masturbation with the same negativity as men (and especially heterosexual men).

An interesting clinical tidbit to add some perspective: When women seek me out for help with masturbation issues, it's usually because they want to have more or better orgasms. When men seek me out for advice about masturbation issues, they usually fear they are having too many orgasms.

I don't believe in "too much" but I definitely believe in "using masturbation as an escape mechanism." There is a significant difference between the two: a socially functional, healthy person may masturbate repeatedly through the day without problems. On the other hand, you could masturbate only once a day and it could still represent a problem. Sex can never be judged as an isolated event; its healthfulness is contingent on whether it fits into your life in a balanced and sane way.

Karl S., a single professional in his mid-30s, was worried that his interest in masturbation was unhealthy. After taking a full sexual history, I concurred. Karl was using masturbation as an escape from problems that were steadily looming larger, threatening his future both socially and professionally. In high school and college, Karl was a friendly, social guy who played sports with friends and went out regularly. Now he was living in an unfamiliar city and working at a high-stress job that required lots of overtime just to remain competitive. By the time he got home at night, he was worn out. He had developed a routine of logging onto the Internet while heating something for dinner, then eating while he browsed the Web for sexual entertainment. By the time he finished his meal, he was hot and bothered and completely obsessed with his on-line sexplay. When he got to a point where he needed relief, he masturbated and went to bed, only to wake up and repeat the cycle the next day. Because he was new in town and didn't know anyone but his work colleagues, who were mostly married, on weekends he stayed in, sometimes spending all his free hours on porn and chat sites. He was spending hundreds of dollars a week on his habit, and beginning to accumulate debt paying for all the on-line sex-workers he chatted with. He was disgusted with himself — the more ashamed he felt, the more he withdrew from people. On a few occasions he got so down on himself, he called in sick to work rather than face the world — and, of course, ended up spending his days off glued to the screen, chatting with sex-workers.

The solution for Karl was to break what was becoming a very troubling and ultimately self-destructive cycle. The more he masturbated, the less he wanted to cope with the world; the poorer his skills at coping with the world, the more he wanted to masturbate to relieve the tension and numb his mind. I suggested that he revise his approach, not by going cold-turkey (which is only seldom effective) but by taking control over his behavioral patterns. As a first step, I recommended that he schedule his masturbation so that he felt he was doing it when he honestly wanted to, and not because he was avoiding his real-world responsibilities. To start, he had to budget his time and expenses for on-line adventure. To help him break the habit, he had to stop hitting the computer first thing when he got home. Going on-line would be a reward after he ate, did laundry, paid bills, or any other chores he typically avoided. Step by step, one small behavioral change at a time, Karl began to focus on the long-neglected parts of his life and imposed a schedule on his play-time, with a strict curfew every night. He began going to the gym regularly, accepted invitations from co-workers he would have blown off before, started going out on weekends, and slowly became the man he used to be. It took him almost a year, during which he backslid and broke his resolutions more than once, but gradually, he emerged from his obsessive sexual fugue and regained his self-respect.

If Karl had come to me saying he masturbated five times a day but was happy, adjusted, functioning, my approach would have been completely different. I would have told him he didn't need therapy. It's a myth that frequent masturbation is a gateway to sexual addiction or psychological problems. There is no evidence whatsoever that people who masturbate regularly become obsessed with it, or need more and crazier masturbation to feel satisfied. Those who have positive sexual self-esteem generally experience masturbation as a warm, fun experience and feel satisfied and complete afterwards. They can repeat the experience as often as they wish, with positive results.

On the other hand, people who are sexually conflicted are the ones at greatest risk of becoming obsessive or compulsive about masturbation. Sometimes they are simply so nervous and over-wrought about their sexuality (or sexual identity) that their sexual impulses are neurotic and malformed. They may lead secret lives in which they indulge in every guilty pleasure they can imagine. They may go on binges — during which they lose all self-control — followed by purges during which they deny and punish themselves. They may have underlying stresses or compulsive tendencies that express themselves sexually (for example, my clinical experience has shown that people with Obsessive Compulsive

Disorder or Attention Deficit Disorder often are OCD or ADD in their sexual behaviors as well).

In all cases, when someone spirals out of control it isn't the fault of the masturbation itself. My clinical experience has repeatedly shown that people who feel comfortable and relaxed about touching themselves are more likely to exert sexual moderation than people who think genitals are dirty or that sexual pleasure is a sin. The more deeply sexually inhibited the client, the more likely he or she is to be compulsive and self-destructive in their sexual behaviors and fantasies.

Alfred M., a man in his mid-40s, told me he occasionally wept after masturbation because he was so disappointed in himself for giving in to his urges. Masturbation had ruined his life. To him, sex was one of life's dirty necessities, like evacuating the bowels. He hated himself for needing to do it but grudgingly accepted that, without it, his internal tension was unbearable. Although heterosexual, he stopped dating seriously years earlier and, on the whole, avoided any form of intimacy with women. Because Alfred never got the satisfaction he needed, he lived in a near-constant state of frustration and mental anguish. By the time he finally saw a sex therapist, Alfred had grown to hate his genitals for causing him so much grief. He was contemplating castration to bring a final end to all his problems. He had found a disreputable doctor on the Internet who was willing to perform the procedure in secret. He just wanted a one-time session with me to hear my opinion.

My opinion was that he had to deal with his low self-esteem before he made the final decision to irreversibly change his life. The larger the picture I was able to develop of Alfred's life, the more I understood the scope of his problems. His mother had been a deeply religious, stern matron, also cold, narcissistic, and verbally abusive. She punished him severely for small infractions, including whipping him with a belt and locking him in a closet. His father was a hollow shell of a man, too intimidated by his wife to help his son. When he was in high school Alfred lost control of the car he was driving, killing his high school sweetheart, a guilt he always still carried with him. Alfred grew up to be a classic underachiever, an overly polite man who was much smarter and better educated than his position in life suggested. Deep down, he was an angry, frightened, deeply wounded man, and perhaps the most difficult and challenging client I've worked with. I acknowledged that he was in pain, and for good reasons, but I didn't think self-mutilation would make him feel any better about himself.

Alfred worked with me, on and off, for almost four years. At times he would vanish and I'd fear the worst but he would return again, ready to push a little further. Working at his pace, I helped him to see that disfigurement was not the solution to emotional conflicts about sex. There were no miracles for Alfred but after three years, he was finally able to find some good things in his life and in himself. Most importantly, he had stopped blaming all his miseries in life on his masturbation and genitals and was now trying to improve himself on several fronts: going to the gym, tentatively dating, and going back to school so he could get a better job.

Anxiety about sex can radically influence a person's life. Exactly how it will play out varies according to individual psychology and circumstances. I've seen a thousand permutations in my practice. I've worked with troubled people who became compulsively promiscuous or led secret double lives — one in which they act and appear completely ordinary, and another where they engage in risky sexual adventures with strangers. I've seen the other extreme, where someone vows to be abstinent because sex feels too complicated and not satisfying enough to make it worth the anguish.

As I occasionally tell clients, "Anxiety is the opposite of sexy." Emotional conflicts thwart a range of sexual responses, from blocking our ability to get aroused to impacting our performance with partners. I believe this concept reaches right into our biology. I think of negative emotions — guilt, fear, shame, disgust, internal conflict — as a massive organic filter through which sexual responses must pass. The more intense those feelings, the more difficult it is for the body and brain to function in harmony. The "happy" brain chemistry of sex is fighting the chemicals released by stress. Muscles which should be relaxing are tensing. Whereas people who are relaxed are assisting their brain in doing its sexual business, people who can't relax are ultimately most likely to be left feeling unsatisfied. It may even cause some of them to crave more and more intensity or experiences just to achieve a simulacrum of the pleasure that balanced people derive from sex. It has been the rule, not the exception, in my clinical practice that the people who make the most disturbingly risky, unhealthy behavioral choices are invariably the ones who are at psychological war in their minds over their sexual identity. They are also the ones who seem to have the most issues and complexes about masturbation, and similarly seem to get the least pleasure out of the act.

In emotionally balanced, socially-adjusted and reasonably physically healthy people, there really is no upper limit on the number of times a day one may safely masturbate. The time to stop is when it stops feeling good; if your genitals start to feel raw, if it's exhausting you, it's common sense to give yourself some time to recover before doing it again. Most typically, high frequency of masturbation simply means a strong sex drive and a robust appetite. On the other hand, if masturbation interferes with or diminishes the quality of your daily life — your ability to socialize, your ability to have intimacy, your ability to focus on work — then it stops being a harmless pleasure and becomes a potentially self-destructive behavior pattern. But the biggest health risk factor related to masturbation seems to be when you do NOT masturbate. Given all the proven benefits of orgasm, failure to masturbate during times when you don't have a partner may reduce your lifespan, speed up your aging process, and contribute to a range of health problems, including heart conditions and immunological disorders.

Finally, as with all sexual behaviors, if you notice a significant change in your pattern of masturbation (if you suddenly start doing it much more than before, or find your interest dwindling to nothing), it is a red flag that something more serious may be going on inside. Ebbs and flows in desire are natural to the cycles of life, but rapid and unexplained (i.e., you aren't pregnant, you aren't in menopause, etc.) changes in sexual behavior are symptomatic of depression, hormonal imbalances, diabetes, and other conditions.

Is Masturbation Really Good For You?

Since masturbation and orgasm instantly stimulate positive change throughout the human organism, masturbating to climax is quite simply the best total wellness exercise one can perform. None of the daily grooming and health rituals we all are taught to do (brushing our teeth, combing our hair, showering) serve the vital purposes of the old-fashioned orgasm. I'll discuss the numerous organic benefits in detail in the section on orgasm but suffice to say, as I so often do, an orgasm a day keeps the doctor away.

As noted earlier, masturbation is our biology's way of preparing us for adult sexuality. It is also our testing ground for skills that will ultimately build to a satisfying sex life in adulthood.

We learn five critical sexual behavioral skills through masturbation:

1. How to produce a state of arousal
2. How to pace sexual pleasure
3. How to enhance sexual pleasure
4. How to delay orgasm
5. How to have an orgasm

Additionally, masturbation teaches us to be comfortable handling our genitals, a key ingredient in a complete sex life. Masturbation is useful in childhood as way of relearning our natural relationship with our bodies after potty training, a time when most parents impress on their children that, by association with urination and elimination, the genital and anal regions are offensive.

Since all of us are potty trained, it's inevitable that many, if not most of us, grow up to believe the whole area is dirty; and since we are all subject to the advice and attitudes of authority figures who tell us that masturbation is bad and that genitals are shameful, forbidden zones, in response to these messages, masturbation often changes from an unselfconscious act to something a child is at least vaguely aware is bad or wrong. Depending on how intensely bad they believe it to be, they may delay or avoid masturbation into adulthood. In some rare cases, early childhood trauma (whether from potty training gone terribly wrong or from child abuse), can permanently damage sex drive and suppress all desire to masturbate.

People who are comfortable with their own genitals tend to be similarly relaxed with their partners' genitals. Knowing that certain spots in and around your genitals are more sensitive than others; knowing what kind of a sensation you crave on your penis or clitoris; knowing which other parts of your body are sensitive to touch all promote an adult's ability to receive and to give satisfying sex. In my practice, I've observed that adults who cannot bear to touch their own genitals, or who believe genitals are dirty, make a lot of excuses to rationalize what are irrational feelings. They set strict boundaries on what "should" or "should not" feel right and have a lot of rules about sex that they make their partners obey — whether it's how often they believe one "should" have intimacy or the types of sexual intimacy one "should" indulge in.

Linda R., a slim, serious women in her early 40s, came to me out of sheer desperation. After thirteen years of marriage, her husband was threatening to leave because he couldn't stand their sex life anymore. She had seen a range of doctors who had examined her and given her pills and patches and creams but nothing had worked. She didn't think I could help her but she was at her wits end.

It took a while to win her trust but finally, through tears, she told me that she had been molested and digitally penetrated by her grandfather when she was five. When she first told her mother about it, she was called a liar and punished. A few months later, he was caught in another child's room. Then all hell broke loose. Linda was dragged in and out of courts to testify against him. To this day, some of her relatives still accuse her of destroying the family.

Linda couldn't think about sex without getting sad. She hated touching herself. She said she felt numb down there but when I asked how she knew for sure if she hadn't experimented, she admitted she didn't. She had baroque methods of toileting and showering, designed to ensure her hand never actually came into contact with the skin of her genitals. She loved her husband "on a higher plane." On those rare occasions when she allowed him intimacy, she "died inside." From the minute he touched her thigh, she tensed and expected pain. The only way she could endure it was by clamping her eyes shut and imagining herself floating above the bed, watching.

Linda had more rules about sexual contact than a chicken has feathers. It could only take place in the bedroom, only after a certain hour in the evening, the lights had to be turned off, it had to be done in silence, and she had a list of places she didn't want her husband to touch, another one for all the acts she would not do, another for how long they could do any one act. When I inquired whether they ever had oral sex, she said, "I don't like him messing around down there." She also admitted she was revolted at the thought of putting his penis in her mouth. To her, genitals were dirty, smelly, ugly and embarrassing parts of the body.

Linda's early experience of trauma had so tragically derailed normal sexual development that, at age 42, she was as innocent as a child about her own body. In order to overcome her fears, Linda was going to have to step outside her comfort zone and finally come to terms with her genitals. The prospect horrified her so much that she didn't come back to see me for nearly two months. When she did, though, she was committed to working on her issues, and did so courageously. Linda will never be exactly the person she might have been without the sexual trauma in her life but it was a glorious victory when she finally began to derive genuine pleasure from her genitals.

At What Ages Do People Start and Stop Masturbating?

Onset of masturbation is too individual to quantify. We know that humans are born sexual. Indeed, we know humans are sexual even before birth, though we have yet to determine how early in its life an embryo responds to erotic stimuli. Research has shown that the male fetus experiences erections in the womb. We also have proof that the fetus is aware when its parents have intercourse and responds with excitement (increased heart-rate) to the adults' orgasms. So given that we are aware of sexual stimuli even before birth, it's safe to assume that we all naturally continue sexual development after we leave the womb.

That said, masturbation begins when a series of events collide in childhood — an unpredictable combination of rate of maturity, opportunity and environment, physical condition and body weight, and underlying biology. A parent who has observed a toddler son rubbing himself strangely on objects or a toddler daughter straddling and bouncing on toys may correctly infer that he or she is practicing a very early, usually unconscious type of masturbation. Similarly, boys may go through a phase in ages 2 to 4 when they seem obsessed with holding their genitals or flashing them inappropriately and little girls may lift up their skirts. However alarming this stage may be to their relatives, it usually ends naturally when the children learn social skills.

A combination of genetics and circumstances/environment dictate how soon kids discover that fascinating area between their legs and make the connection between touching it and feeling good. Although there are, of course, exceptions, in general when pre-pubertal children masturbate, it's not in the ways or for the complex emotional and physiological reasons that adults do. Children are not driven by adult body chemistry and hormones, nor do they seek out sex partners (though they may randomly experiment with children their own age as the opportunity arises). Masturbation isn't "goal oriented." They aren't trying to have an orgasm. If we masturbate when we're children, it's because we are biologically disposed to begin the long journey to sexual adulthood through self-experimentation. The simpler explanation, of course, is that when we find something that feels good, we want to do it again.

Adolescent and adult masturbation, as I define it, is when a person can have a complete experience of masturbation: it's when we do it consciously, knowing that if we touch ourselves not only will it feel good, but that we may experience an orgasm as a result. We may use masturbation for psychological reasons — to comfort ourselves when we feel sad, to add excitement to the day, to compensate for the lack of a partner, and so on. We may use masturbation for physiological ones too, to relieve sexual tension or stress. Whatever our reasons, masturbation in teens and adults is usually deliberate. (Conversely, teens and adults who continue to masturbate unconsciously or chronically as children do are, in my opinion, generally suffering from psycho-sexual or developmental disorders that thwarted them from maturing to a balanced and adult model of sexual behavior.)

From my clinical experience, I've noted that most males seem to start consciously masturbating at puberty, when their penis is growing to adult size and they are developing hair and deeper voices. This is usually between 12 and 14, but I've talked to men who began maturing at 10 or 11; and others who, though fully mature, didn't consciously masturbate until they were 17 or 18. It has been my observation that girls more commonly start masturbating later than boys, often in their mid-teens to early college age. Age of menstruation — which is a signal that adult hormones are now coursing through a girl's body — is roughly the age when most girls can have a complete masturbatory experience. Still, many girls delay self-experimentation.

I believe that female masturbation would naturally track male masturbation "in the wild" but we don't live in the wild. In the world we live in, sex and sexuality are exceedingly complicated for women, both culturally and physically. (I'll go into this in depth in the section on Female Sexuality.) In brief, while adults may choose to have sex and then work on getting aroused, in our teens we are far more likely to be guided by our genitals. When boys and young men have spontaneous erections, they quickly realize that they can relieve the swelling by manual stimulation. The subject of masturbation is eternal fodder for locker room jokes. Between their unmistakable physical arousal and some measure of acceptance that it's normal for boys to be horny, I believe boys develop a stronger and more easily studied pattern of masturbation than girls.

For better or worse, teen girls do not have obviously visible signs of excitement. Their organs do not suddenly balloon in their underpants, and if they grow a little moist, no one (including the girls themselves) may know. And whereas boys are allowed to be crude hellions, girls are expected to be sweet misses. They are pushed to see themselves as non-sexual and praised for being virginal. I believe these attitudes slow girls down, distort their perception of their own sexual identity, and present obstacles to female sexual satisfaction later in life.

Frequency and intensity of masturbation both cycle throughout our lives, along with our hormones and our circumstances. Whether partnered or single, it is normal for a person's sexual desire to wax and wane throughout his or her life and for masturbatory habits to follow those natural cycles. Newly partnered couples may abandon masturbation for partnered sex in their honeymoon phase, and return to it when sexual contact in the partnership declines. Some will use it as an adjunct throughout their lives. Some use it to compensate during periods apart. It is extremely common for pregnant women to avoid or defer sex, and just as common for their husbands to compensate with masturbation. Negative life events — job loss, illness, depression — typically diminish libido. Positive life events — career success, new relationships, vacations — typically boost it.

Overall, the drive to have an orgasm diminishes with age, and so does the frequency of masturbation, but if you take reasonably good care of your sexual health, and let doctors offer you the best in current sexual healthcare, one may masturbate until the end of one's life. I've worked with clients in their 60s and 70s who were still going strong. After the age of 80, sexual performance and drive is difficult to quantify. Generally, the people who were libidinous and sexually active in their youths and middle ages, will continue to want and need sex in old age, while those who were not very sexual in the first place may lose all desire for intimacy.

Just as masturbation is the first sexual behavior we explore it is often the last one we perform. When we outlive our partners, are too feeble to enjoy sex with a partner, or face other obstacles of old age, the ability to masturbate is often the last type of sex people enjoy.

⋙ Chapter Two ⋘

A Brief History of Masturbation

———◄◊►———

Why We Think Something So Right is So Wrong

So why did humans think masturbation was wrong in the first place? For centuries, people have traded stories and myths about how masturbation causes hair to grow on palms, can lead to blindness or will sap your natural vitality. Maybe you've assumed some of those things were true. To set you straight, here's an abbreviated history of the misapprehensions, mistakes and outright quackery that have shaped contemporary ideas about masturbation and orgasm.

Since ancient times, philosophers, thinkers, and religious figures have argued and opined about the morals of masturbation. There are some scant records of cultures which accepted masturbation as a normal act. An ancient Egyptian myth held that the first man and woman were created when the Sun God masturbated them into being. In ancient Sumerian religion, when the god Enki masturbated, his ejaculate flowed to the earth and created the Tigris River.

However, as far back as records go, an honest embrace of masturbation seems to be the exception. Contemporary scientists of every ilk have speculated about why societies heaped such opprobrium upon auto-eroticism. Was it because humans realized there is power in numbers and instinctively tried to ensure that sexual energy was reserved for the only type of sex which carries the chance of impregnation? Or because religious movements and societies wished to control and direct sexuality for political or economic purposes? Perhaps people took the Biblical commandment to multiply so literally they felt anything less than a potentially reproductive act was heresy?

I'm tantalized by all the speculation but all we know for sure is that taboos against masturbation seem to be as old as humanity itself, yet — in the light of modern science — no one can make a rational case to explain why. Indeed, the entire case against masturbation is a long, absurdist history of misinformation, religious duplicity, and prejudice piled on top of quackery.

For most of human history, attitudes toward masturbation were either religious or philosophic in nature, and followed the teachings of clergy and moralists. But in the first decade of the 18th century, a pamphlet was printed which declared that masturbation was physically harmful too. Its title: *Onania; or, The Heinous Sin of Self Pollution, and all its Frightful Consequences, in both SEXES Considered, with Spiritual and Physical Advice to those who have already injured themselves by this abominable practice. And seasonable Admonition to the Youth of the nation of Both SEXES.*

Published anonymously ca. 1712-1718, *Onania* was an instant bestseller. The pamphlet likely was written as an advertising brochure for the "cures" it recommended, "Strengthening Tincture" and "Prolific Powder." But the reading public could not get enough of the ghoulish descriptions and illustrations of the horrors certain to attend those who rubbed their own genitals. Their organs rotted; they went mad; they turned into hermaphrodites; and worse. And within a few decades, Western perceptions of masturbation shifted from religious/moral opinion to something that sounded medical and therefore authoritative.

(I've always felt sorry for poor, misunderstood Biblical Onan, whose name became enshrined in our cultural lexicon as a synonym for masturbation. In the Bible, Onan was actually chastised for defiance, not masturbation: he defied God's order to impregnate his dead brother's wife. Moreover, he did not masturbate: he penetrated her but then pulled out of her and let his sperm drip to the ground.)

In 1758, seeking to rectify some of the most ludicrous claims forwarded in *Onania*, and to issue a genuinely medical opinion on the subject, a Swiss doctor named Samuel-Auguste Tissot (1728-1797) produced one of the most influential volumes of his age. *Onanism: Or a Treatise Upon the Disorders produced by Masturbation: Or, the Dangerous Effects of Secret and Excessive Venery*, claimed to scientifically analyze masturbation.

In it, Tissot asserted that semen was an essential body oil. He believed that if you lost too much of your oil, you would dry up and become vulnerable to diseases. He claimed that losing an ounce of semen was the equivalent of losing 40 ounces of blood (2 pints). Doing Tissot's math, if you masturbated three times a day, you lost over half the blood in your body. Thus Tissot concluded that masturbation had frighteningly debilitating effects on your health, among them blindness and insanity.

That Tissot had no valid proof of his theories did not diminish their legitimacy in the eyes of his peers. In the 18th century, physicians still thought that human health was ruled by "the four humors," that blood-letting cured most diseases, and that you could diagnose a person's health by the bumps on his skull (phrenology). Metaphysics, alchemy, magical thinking, pharmacological follies and charlatanism — what Levi-Strauss termed "the shamanistic complex" — dominated the scientific landscape. Scientific study as we know it today would not exist for another 100 years. (Neither would the legal concept of medical malpractice, which was not formulated until the late 19th century.)

Most significantly, Tissot's assertions recapitulated the opinions clergy had been expressing for centuries. What had long been viewed as sin was now regarded as medically unsafe. Churches and the public at large embraced this justification of their religious beliefs. Throughout Europe, moralists and clergy who had formerly preached an anti-masturbation doctrine based on spiritual considerations (such as the threat of burning in hell for "self-abuse"), now used Tissot's study as solid evidence of the grave risks people faced if they indulged their auto-erotic lusts. Tissot's work was considered ground-breaking and its science was unquestioned, even among his scientific and intellectual peers. German philosopher, Immanuel Kant, was inspired by Tissot to voice his own condemnations of masturbation in *The Metaphysics of Morals.*

Tissot's work set the template for the future scientific and med-ico-forensic establishment's view of masturbation. Throughout the 18th and 19th centuries, and well into the 20th, the prevailing scholarly and scientific opinion of masturbation was that it was risky behavior and should be prevented to preserve public health. Religious leaders of every stripe — along with an astonishing num-ber of reputable doctors and psychiatrists — set about trying to cure people of the urge to touch themselves. But it was the rising tide of charlatanism, moving in tandem with the development of modern Western medicine, that made the 19th century a particu-larly loathsome and dark period in the history of human sexuality.

In the U.S., Sylvester Graham (1784-1851), founder of the Ameri-can Vegetarian society and an ordained Presbyterian minister, became a vigorous proponent of a "cure" for masturbation. In tracts, pamphlets, sermons and speeches, Graham advocated chastity and celibacy, insisting that all men should remain virgins until they were 30. Even when married, Graham advised that men limit sexual relations to once per month. These measures, Gra-ham believed, were necessary to maintain good moral character and overall health. In 1829, Graham revealed that he had invented a miraculous and wholesome bread that cured lust. In the true American entrepreneurial spirit, he made a fortune marketing "Graham bread" to the credulous masses who believed their lives depended on denying themselves orgasms. Today we know that the bread didn't cure anything but a moment's hunger. Still Gra-ham's social influence rose as his financial fortunes climbed. (By the way, these days we call his bread a Graham cracker and the manufacturers follow an improved recipe. You may eat your pie crust and have your lust too.) Graham was also famous for his "electric bed," a contraption which allegedly cured impotence.

John Harvey Kellogg (1852-1943), a devout Seventh Day Adventist and a medical doctor, was arguably the oddest and most sadistic sex crank America ever produced. Born a year after Graham died, Kellogg subscribed whole-heartedly to his predecessor's ideologies and, like Graham, vehemently opposed sex for pleasure. Kellogg devoted himself to curing masturbation, which he believed resulted in atrophied testicles. He also championed the use of enemas and purgatives in the belief that the more you poop, the healthier you become. Kellogg perceived the human body as a kind of primordial swamp of pollutants, with only fragile resources of strength and vitality. In his view, the anus was to be regularly flushed of its poisons, while semen was a precious commodity to be preserved at all costs. Like Graham, Kellogg believed he had invented a superior comestible: his food would cure people of masturbation and make them have more bowel movements too. And so America was introduced to Kellogg's Cornflakes. Which, of course, did not work either, but which many people found a tasty and convenient new breakfast option.

For those genteel ladies and gentlemen who could afford more sophisticated treatments, Kellogg's famous Battle Creek Sanatarium offered masturbation aversion therapy by draconian methods. Kellogg and his clinical staff set about genitally tormenting and mutilating clients to engender what they considered a healthy terror of sex. Using electro- and hydro-therapies, genital cages and traps, Kellogg's staff tortured clients for their own good.

The use of electronic gadgets to "cure" sexual disorders had been around since the 1770s, when galvanic "cures" were offered by quacks and legitimate doctors alike. Electro-therapy for sex problems gained further credibility in the 19th century, when prolific author, surgeon and respected neurologist, George M. Beard (1839-1883) claimed he had suffered "neurasthenia" (believed at the time to be a sexual disorder which caused men to be weak, tired, and impotent) as a young man and "cured" himself with electricity. Because of Beard's excellent scientific reputation, electro-therapy became a standard medical treatment both to stimulate better erections with mild levels of shock and to discourage men from masturbating with excruciatingly high levels.

Electroshock to the genitals was by no means the cruelest method of preventing masturbation. In his publication, *Treatments for Self Abuse and Its Effects*, Kellogg advocated circumcision for boys and chemical clitorectomy with carbolic acid for girls. Not only did he believe in mutilating children, he also believed the genital mutilations should be performed as painfully as possible to instill a permanent terror in patients so they would never want to touch their genitals again. Kellogg and his contemporaries may be credited with the popularization of circumcision in America, something I'll discuss in more depth in the section on male sexual health.

We may laugh at Kellogg and Graham today but, like Tissot, they influenced the leaders and thinkers of their day. Horace Greeley, sometimes called the father of the Republican Party, was so persuaded by Sylvester Graham's theories, he kept an apartment separately from his wife to ensure he did not weaken or damage his health by overindulging in Mrs. Greeley's charms.

Throughout the 1800s and into the mid-1900s, charismatic charlatans and money-hungry doctors throughout the Western World and its colonies continued to cash in on the anti-masturbation craze by selling snake oil and sadistic appliances to the masses. Most of these devices operated on the principle that aversion therapy — teaching men to associate fear and pain with genital stimulation — would put an end to masturbation. Among the numerous devices manufactured to cure self-stimulation: a "Penis Cooling Device," invented by Frank Orth (1893); the Stephenson Spermatic Truss (1876); a saw-toothed steel penis ring to prevent erection (1908); a leather and steel penis "corset," invented by a Dr. Fleck (1931). These and dozens of other types of cages and chastity contraptions were routinely used on boys and men, not only in the spas and clinics run by charlatans, but in hospitals and mental wards throughout Europe and North America, where psychiatrists eagerly applied themselves to the task of "curing" male masturbation by causing intense pain to their genitals.

Even as some sex doctors and quacks worked feverishly on remedies for masturbation, others devoted themselves to improving male virility. Strange but true, doctors at the time did not see any contradiction between, on one hand, trying to make men give up masturbation and, on the other, trying to give them better erections. Wedded as they were to the RM, they believed that erections had a single biological function: to impregnate women. Any pleasure from the act was a secondary feature, a reward for doing their duty. They also believed the stronger the erection, the better the sperm, and the healthier the child it produced. Thus, men and their doctors alike worried mightily about the quality of men's erections. Since the RM was the only legitimate form of sex, the occurrence of impotence was far more devastating to men of this period than we can imagine. Erections defined masculinity: without one, men were made to feel they had no purpose in life.

The German doctor, Carl von Graef, was one of the most successful mid-19th century quacks to exploit the Victorian male's fears of erectile dysfunction. After spending time in Spain, where he learned about the native herbs Yerba Santa and Yerba Rheub, von Graef announced he had discovered the ultimate remedy for all male sexual dysfunctions. Calling his yerba-based formula "The Great Spanish Remedy," and setting up offices in New York City, the Von Graef Company manufactured and marketed "trochees" (lozenges) in the late 19th century, advising that the medicine could either be swallowed whole or dissolved onto the male member. Their lushly illustrated pamphlets claimed that von Graef's trochees cured impotence, increased virility, stopped nocturnal emissions, AND eliminated the urge to masturbate. All at the same time.

Fast on von Graef's heels was the American doctor and entrepreneur, John R. Brinkley (1885 - 1942). It was Brinkley's special theory that glands removed from goat testicles could be implanted into humans to cure a wide range of unrelated ailments, including impotence, dementia, lung disease, tumors, and (my favorite) flatulence. With his prodigious gift for self-promotion, Brinkley initiated an aggressive direct-mail campaign, hiring an ad man who provided an appealing slogan that promised to turn every man into "the ram that am with every lamb." Brinkley soon became known as "the goat gland king," and broadened his insane surgical experiments towards women. Indeed, it was his dismally unsuccessful treatment of a woman — who received a transplant of goat glands in her ovaries — that first brought him to the attention of the American Medical Association.

There were so many charlatans promising cures for masturbation along with drugs, surgeries, and painful treatments for impotence that no one could hope to make an accurate count of them all. There was a Dr. Serge Voronoff, who grafted monkey testicles into men in the 1920s. In 1914, a Dr. G. Frank Lydston experimented with grafting human testicles, using himself as a guinea pig and implanting the testicles of a dead convict in his own scrotum. The resident physician at San Quentin prison, a Dr. L. L. Stanley, inspired by the work of Voronoff, performed testicle grafting experiments similar to Lydston's, and later injected over 650 of the unwitting convicts in his care with solutions made from the testicles of goats, rams, boars and bucks.

Throughout the 19th and early 20th century, penny papers and cheap magazines were chock-a-block with deceptive ads by shady characters claiming their snake-oil solved all male sexual health problems. Millions of advertisements and pamphlets — often designed to look like genuine medical brochures — were mailed to unsuspecting consumers throughout the United States. Some entrepreneurs — such as John Brinkley — became fabulously wealthy from their quack remedies; others were small-time con artists who scraped by selling their cures at carnivals and fairs. Indeed, self-promoters and cranks continue to exploit the American public's sexual ignorance today as well, though now instead of snake oil, they hawk "penis enhancers."

Attitudes towards female masturbation and response has a much quirkier history. For one, prior to the 19th century, women's health was a low priority to doctors, in large part because women were second-class citizens, economically, socially and otherwise. Female sexual health was looked down on as unpleasant, untidy, and disagreeable work, unfit for high-minded physicians — an attitude which many women complain still prevails today. Neither they nor their problems received the serious attention that men received; physicians did not expend any energy on developing theories or treatments for female complaints. Prior to the 20th century, physicians were health consultants: patients never removed their clothes. They explained their symptoms, physicians diagnosed the disease and wrote them prescriptions or recommended surgeries. Hands-on contact with patients was largely reserved for trained surgeons, who might not meet a patient until he was lying on their operating table.

Finally, and perhaps most importantly, until the 20th century, the medical establishment accepted doctrinal teachings on female sexuality as a fundamental truth. Women were not by nature sexual: women were either virgins or whores. Virgins were authentic, honest, women; whores were diseased compatriots of Satan. Even when they married, women did not enjoy sex: they only enjoyed making their husband's happy through their obedience. Thus cures for female masturbation were barely necessary: only very depraved, and usually insane, women had such impulses.

So while men consulted physicians for their sexual problems, for thousands of years, midwives served as women's doctors, healers and sexual confidantes. Midwives tended to any and all sexual health issues women had, from menstruation to menopause and everything in between. According to a number of sources, midwives were the first to offer women relief in the form of what we today call a "happy ending." The "pelvic massage" (or "vaginal massage") was a standard folk medicine remedy for women suffering symptoms of "female hysteria," including symptoms of PMS, tension, anxiety and, of course, sheer sexual frustration.

In the 19th century, the role and reputation of midwives dramatically changed. With the growing medicalization of sexuality, and the flowering of medicine as an exact science, came the dawning realization that female sexual health was important to a stable society. Scientists and doctors who previously ignored women's sexuality now began to take an interest in all the conditions formerly treated by midwives.

Jean-Martin Charcot (1825-1893) was among the first to focus his considerable intellect on the sexual and mental health problems of women. One of the most renowned figures in 19th century European medicine, and the most highly regarded and innovative neurologists of his time, his early theories about female sexuality were regarded worshipfully by the talented and brilliant students who studied under him, among them Sigmund Freud.

Charcot, Freud, and other eminent sexologists of the 19th century saw themselves as humanists: theirs was a more compassionate, clinical perspective than the medieval point of view that women with strong sex drives were Satanic witches who deserved persecution, incarceration and death. I believe in their good intentions, however their science on female sexuality was as flawed and absurd as many of the crank theorists who preceded them.

They still operated on the assumptions that, first, sex drive is a male phenomenon and, second, that the RM (Reproductive Model) of sex is the only "right" or "normal" type of sex. Healthy, normal women did not need or want sex because they didn't experience the urge for sexual pleasure the way men do. Women who engaged in non-RM sex were "hypersexual," a neurological disorder. Masturbation, lesbianism or promiscuity were symptoms of hypersexuality. Conversely, women who avoided physical contact, who didn't submit to their husbands' requests for sex, or who complained of daily aches, pains, headaches, faintness, anxiety, or mood swings were diagnosed as "hysteric." Female hysteria was a threat to population growth, to the personal happiness of men, and thus to society in general. In the belief that women are passive vessels for men's pleasure, they set about trying to fix those vessels so that women would be restored to their ideal model of an obedient woman who has sex with her husband out of a higher sense of duty to family and nation.

"Hysteria" as a diagnosis for women who behaved badly — and particularly those who seemed to enjoy sex — is as old as Western culture. Hysteria (from the Greek "hustera" = uterus) was first coined by Hippocrates, the ancient Greek philosopher (460 BC – ca. 370 BC), who believed that the uterus wandered around the female body and, in some women, rose to their chest and strangled them, causing them to go mad. In the second century (AD), the physician Galen offered a more descriptive definition: hysteria was a "disease" suffered by excessively libidinous women who were denied sex.

Using research he gathered in the mental wards of the Salpêtrière Hospital in Paris, Charcot updated these traditional theories of female hysteria, claiming he now had verifiable proof. Charcot's research was the platform for Freud's expanded work on the subject. A rapidly growing industry of physicians, psychiatrists and quacks — often indiscernible from one another — now set out to cure women who did not conform to the idealized model of femininity. By 1860, doctors were claiming that a full one quarter of all women suffered from sexual disorders. That was the bad news. The good news was that they had cures.

"Female troubles" turned out to be an economic boon for the medical establishment, which used its growing political and social power to drive midwives out of business as unqualified competition. New laws limited midwives' services, relegating them primarily to attending or assisting at births. Their other traditional functions were now replaced by sexologists, psychologists, obstetricians and gynecologists.

With the growing scientific focus on the uterus and the womb, surgeons also set about perfecting another technique first developed in ancient Greece: the hysterectomy. Although most doctors then as now used the surgery to treat cancer, medical historians have numerously catalogued examples of 19th and 20th century doctors who performed hysterectomies to "cure" over-sexed women. By removing all or part of their reproductive organs, they believed women would calm down and become more sexually obedient.

A much more popular cure for female hysteria, however, was the newly medicalized pelvic massage. Although midwives had provided this service for over 1600 years, doctors now endeavored to "cure" hysteria by inducing "hysterical paroxyms" (i.e., orgasms). Strange but true, the same generations of doctors who tortured children and men for touching themselves, and who did not believe that women should experience sexual lust, continued to subscribe to the practice of pelvic massage. As doctors saw it (or at least, as they told themselves), hysteria was a bona fide neurological disorder, proven by the finest minds in Europe. Rubbing their patients' genitals had nothing to do with sex.

Not surprisingly, masturbatory services for women disguised as health remedies was a lucrative business throughout the 19th century. Rich ladies of the upper classes clamored for the curative services available at elite sanitariums and spas throughout Europe. The legendary hot springs of Bath (England) offered private treatment baths to relax the nerves of their neurotic female clientele. Fed by the hot springs, water jets were strategically positioned to deliver hydrotherapeutic thrills to the bather's groin, bringing her to "therapeutic" release.

Private doctors advertised more affordable treatments. Their method was simple and effective: they used their hands. Pelvic massages became so fashionable, that they created some unusual challenges to the doctors who performed them. For one, all the rubbing and thrusting was wearing out their wrists. For another, many Victorian doctors were embarrassed by the procedure; some felt it was unsanitary to touch their patients' genitals. Rather than forego this profitable treatment, however, medical inventors found a technological solution. In the 1870s, the first clockwork dildo was invented, followed a few years later by an electro-mechanical version. These precursors to today's motorized toys allowed doctors to induce orgasms efficiently and clinically, sparing them both repetitive stress injuries and the affront to their fastidious sensibilities.

While these stories may seem ridiculous to us now, it's hard to fault people back then for not knowing what we know today. Far more disturbing is that beliefs about the harmfulness of masturbation persisted long after educated people knew the early theories were so flawed as to be preposterous. The medical, forensic, and psychiatric communities remained stolidly in agreement that masturbation was a disease they could treat, even though there was no proof that it was a disease, and abundant proof that none of their cures worked. Throughout the 20th century, women and men were still being operated on, forced to submit to aversion therapy, involuntarily hospitalized in mental wards, and required to take medications, all in aid of "curing" them of masturbatory and other non-RM sexual behaviors. Boys and girls were warned that it would endanger their health and ruin their social prospects. Athletes were told they would lose muscle mass and energy if they indulged. Married people were chastised if they didn't reserve all their sexual energies for intercourse. Adults who admitted to masturbating could be diagnosed as pathological.

Beginning in the 1940s, helping professionals finally began to question the assumptions that had been unquestioned since Tissot's time. With the 1948 publication of Alfred Kinsey's scientific study of human sexuality, we had, for the first time, reliable evidence that the RM was only one type of a wide range of consensual adult behavior. Kinsey proved that so-called aberrant sex acts, including masturbation, were common and even beneficial expressions of human sex drive. With those data, Kinsey permanently changed the discourse on masturbation.

Still, the cultural status quo of sexual ignorance was only marginally improved, in part because of the massive push-back against Kinsey's nonconformist assertions. His work was viewed as heretical; his reputation was vilified by pretty much everyone who was invested in the belief that the only right kind of sex was the RM. Meanwhile, phony anti-masturbation cures and aversion therapies continued to trot along at a profitable pace, only now they carried the respectable mantle of approved medicine. Throughout the 1950s, psychiatrists and physicians still used many 19th century techniques to cure known masturbators, along with new psychotropic drugs and psychoanalysis. Needless to say, they were no more successful with their treatments than anyone else.

It was not until 1961 that the American Psychiatric Association, forced by the preponderance of evidence that masturbation could not be cured because it was not a disease, grudgingly removed masturbation from its list of pathologies. This meant that a person could no longer be diagnosed as mentally ill because he or she masturbated. It also meant that APA members could no longer offer to cure masturbation, something which angered many doctors who had been earning a good living offering false hope. Despite the depathologization of masturbation, many doctors continued to believe the behavior was harmful and aberrant. It would take several more decades for the facts about masturbation to emerge from behind the fortress of shame that surrounds the subject. In 2011, we have significant quantities of scientific research which all point to the same conclusion: masturbation is not just normal, it is a healthful practice, and possible a necessary one for good physical and mental health. Public opinion, however, is still in the grip of past anti-masturbatory ideology, myth and legend.

In the absence of free and open dialogue about masturbation, all the myths perpetrated in *Onania* about the dangers of masturbation are still repeated from parents to offspring, and from schoolchild to schoolchild, and, most frustrating of all, occasionally from clergy to congregation and from helping professional to patient. There are people out there who still believe that aversion therapy (severe punishment) for masturbation will cure it; there are those who believe the power of prayer will cast the masturbatory demon out. And most people still feel too ashamed to admit they do it and too embarrassed to ask questions about it. Only seven years ago, in 1994, Dr. Jocelyn Elders was forced to resign as U.S. Surgeon General for stating what every competent doctor knew: masturbation is a normal aspect of human sexuality.

Finally, it's important to note that while most of our official institutions, and the majority of public opinion, held somewhat unified positions against masturbation as a social ill, throughout human history there have always been individuals, groups, and movements (religious and political) who advocated for sexual freedom, who celebrated the body, and whose opinions and attitudes were, in retrospect, visionary in their time. In our time, the door to a new view of masturbation was opened by author and artist Betty Dodson, whose breakthrough book *Sex for One* (first published in 1974) offered the common reader more insights and truths about sexuality than the previous century of science yielded.

⇥ Chapter Three ⇤

Orgasm

———◄◦►———

Afterter masturbation, comes... you. One hopes. This section explores the facts about orgasm as we know them right now. As with all the science in this book, one should expect that new understandings and findings will emerge that help us gain more insights into the mysteries of the body and brain.

First Step to Orgasm: Arousal

Arousal is the first stage of sex: it's the period when your body prepares for a sexual experience.

Most people think arousal begins when they see its visible signs. An erection in males, vaginal wetness in females, hard nipples, faster breathing, increased body heat, sweat, and other changes in our bodies are some of the obvious signs that we are ready for sex. When we are aroused, the sensitivity in our genitals becomes radically heightened. Compare it to how your genitals feel when they are relaxed or when you urinate. We don't yet fully understand how the engorgement of blood in our genitals and the flow of brain chemicals combine to vastly enhance receptivity to stimuli, but we can say at least that genital congestion is a hallmark of arousal.

Although most of us are taught to think that sex "happens down there," brain research and endocrinological data prove that sex neither begins nor ends in the genitals. During arousal, we may feel, on a conscious level, as if our genitals are running the show. In fact, they are more like the stars of the show, grabbing all the glory. But, behind the scenes, a thousand other players work furiously to ensure that the stars' performance will be a success. While the time between when our brains first register an opportunity for sex to when we feel a stirring in our loins may take only seconds, the genitals are actually the last parts of the body to respond in the lightning-fast chain of sexual reactions. Your brain triggers changes in the nervous system, the circulatory system, the cardiovascular system, the reproductive system, muscle groups, and our body's largest organ, our skin, to achieve a successful outcome — and without the cooperation of your entire biological entity, arousal may not occur.

While most of the signs of arousal listed above are reliable indicators of being turned on, sometimes those signs lie. Male and female bodies alike are technically capable of engaging in and completing a sex act, because our brains are adapted to exploit physical opportunities for sex. However if your individual psychology is not on the same page as your body, even a man with an erection or a woman with a moist vagina will not "feel" aroused. For example, a rape victim may have all the physical responses we associate with arousal yet feel revolted and terrified on a conscious level. It is fairly common for people (particularly in adolescence) to experience spontaneous arousal, even getting turned on by things that actually disgust or frighten them. People coerced into sexual slavery or forced prostitution, for example, may be able to perform physically yet experience deep emotional trauma.

Although you can be physically aroused without consent, emotions and psychology dictate whether or not you will enjoy the experience. Conventional models of sexuality often ignore that crucial mind-body connection, placing emphasis instead on the physical responses. But contemporary studies have repeatedly shown that our emotional state is the key to a satisfying experience of sex.

As a clinician, I'm often struck by how changes in attitudes towards sex can transform a person's sexual pleasure and performance level. More often than not, it is a person's emotions about sex that create sexual problems, not their physical health or attributes. Once their conflicts and ambivalence about sex begin to resolve, their dysfunctions diminish and disappear.

How and why it is that emotional reactions to sex are more important to enjoyment than actual sexual function is still open to debate and study. What we do know is that non-consensual sexual contact, no matter how seemingly mild (e.g., unwanted groping), appears to be emotionally harmful in all instances, whether you are three or ninety-three. Its opposite is true as well: if your mind is willing, no matter the type or intensity of the sex, the experience will likely be pleasurable and emotionally harmless. As far as our biologies are concerned, whether it's the RM, oral sex, gay sex, bondage sex, or anything else, sex feels good when our internal, subjective reality believes the circumstances are right.

Conversely, a person can be extremely aroused and not have any visible signs of arousal. For example, a male can feel fully sexually excited yet achieve only a partial erection; and a female's arousal may be difficult to detect if she isn't lubricating heavily. Sometimes the only way of knowing if your partner is aroused is if he or she tells you so.

For these reasons, arousal as a complete mind/body experience is even more difficult to analyze than its physiological components. The full picture of the hows and whys of sexual response continues to elude our understanding, though data are beginning to emerge. Why are some of us frequently aroused while others seldom feel aroused at all? What makes us respond sexually to one thing instead of another? Why is consent so important to arousal? Why are some people turned off by things that turn other people on? Why can't we rationally choose who we will be sexually attracted to? The answers to dozens of questions like these are buried in individual psychology and our DNA. Current genetic research on sex and other emotional and social behaviors offer the intriguing possibility that things we have always assumed were random or accidental are actually the product of genetic heritage, including who we find attractive and how we perform in bed.

What is an Orgasm?

An orgasm is a biological means of relieving sexual and other psychological tensions, and a mechanism to flush natural mood enhancers (endorphins, oxytocin, and vasopressin) through the body. The purposes of these brain "drugs" are still being studied but are known to be crucial to psychological, social and emotional well-being, including our urges for intimacy, bonding, and parenting.

Based on what we already know, it is not unreasonable to argue that orgasms are a factor in the well-being of couples and relationship stability. As noted above, data suggests that the release of sexual hormones as a result of orgasm increases an adult's urge to form closer loving bonds with both partners and children.

OK, but What is an Orgasm Really?

The challenge in defining what an orgasm is, or more properly how it feels, is the same challenge one faces in describing things like "happiness" or "well-being" or even "love." The problem with orgasms is that they don't just feel different depending on who you talk to, they actually are different. Not just physically but emotionally.

Some of us experience orgasm as a slow, steady climb towards an overwhelming state of excitement that suddenly rockets us out of conscious being and into a state of ecstasy. Along with feelings of relief and satisfaction there may also be profound emotions, including passion, romance, love, intimacy, and bonding. Certainly that is how most literature (fiction and non-fiction) describes orgasm. In real life, however, there are always variations.

Some people do not "climb" slowly and steadily towards release but naturally orgasm very quickly. They may climax only minutes (or even seconds) after first feeling aroused. (This is not the same as involuntary orgasm, or premature orgasm, which I'll talk about later in this section.) Some people need lengthy stimulation or foreplay before achieving climax. Some find that foreplay is more exciting than the climax itself. Some enjoy delaying orgasm and lingering in a state of arousal and desire. Some are goal-oriented in their sex and use arousal/foreplay primarily to warm up their muscles and organs. Others (female and male alike) are multi-orgasmic and do not experience "One Big O" but rather have strings of orgasms that may or may not be as powerful as one big one, depending on the individual. Some people howl and writhe from the intensity of an orgasm; others simply gasp. Some people find that an orgasm wakes them up, mentally, physically and spiritually; others just want to roll over and go to sleep.

It is not unusual for an adult to have fantastic orgasms with one partner and mediocre orgasms with another — even when those partners do more or less the same things in bed. What no amount of study can pin down and place on a matrix are the individual emotions and mitigating circumstances which dictate whether sex will be an ecstatic experience or just an experience. For some, that means orgasm in a monogamous context with a familiar, trusted lover. The trust factor, in particular, appears crucial in adult women's ability to fully experience the intensity of sexual pleasure. Still, some people have their best orgasms with strangers. For them, it's the unknown, even the forbidden flavor of a new encounter which produces the most intense erotic responses. Most of us fall in between those ends of the spectrum and find that we can and do enjoy both casual sex and bonded sex.

Occasionally, sexual response can be impacted by seemingly unimportant factors. Ruth F. came to me complaining of chronic inorgasmia. She mentioned that it had always been a struggle for her to enjoy sex in bed. A childhood victim of sexual abuse, she was only able to relax in bed when she wore pajamas. Removing her clothes and relaxing in bed felt like a stressful chore. So I suggested she explore the rest of the house. To our mutual delight, it turned out she had very nice orgasms in the bathroom and other rooms she didn't associate with her early trauma.

There is no single orgasmic ideal to which everyone must attain. Unfortunately, so much of the literature (particularly fiction, but also plenty of sexual advice books) place the emphasis on the fireworks one is supposed to feel. I've spoken with many people who felt perennially disappointed in themselves because their orgasms seemed tepid and unremarkable compared to the orgasms they'd read about in books. They thought everyone but them were having mind-blowing orgasms every time.

One of the key messages I relay to clients is that none of us can have someone else's orgasm: we can only have our own. Working with one's own potential — learning which kinds of sensations, body parts, and activities make you feel most excited and alive, keeping your sex organs healthy, toning your sex-related muscles to improve your performance, feeling spiritually and emotionally connected to your erotic identity and feeling good about where and when you have your orgasm — are the building blocks of great orgasms.

How Long does it Take to Climax & How Long do Orgasms Last?

The amount of time it takes an individual to climax, and the duration of their orgasms, are both variables in the sexual equation. On average, it can take anywhere from under a minute to over an hour to achieve climax, depending on the type of stimulation, the circumstances, the partner (or lack thereof), personal health, and mood.

I've yet to see any proof of a direct correlation between lack of inhibition and speed of orgasm or vice versa. I've worked with extremely sexually inhibited clients who are able to tune out all the negativity during the act of masturbation and bring themselves to orgasm very quickly. I've also worked with self-confident hedonists who can spontaneously jump into a sexual experience and climax quickly. My surmise is that duration of orgasm is more physiological and circumstantial — meaning a combination of individual biology and real-life circumstances (who you are with, what you are doing, where you are).

Some sexual gourmets deliberately deny themselves orgasm, or defer an orgasm, to attenuate their excitement and build very slowly (hours, even days) to a profound sexual tension and anticipation before final release.

Studies in men's health suggest that the average time from arousal to climax in adult males is between 5 and 7 minutes. Once you start to climax, the physiological experience of orgasm can last anywhere from a couple of seconds to a minute. Again, it all depends on your own wiring, whether you are having an optimal sexual experience (i.e., having the kind of sex that turns you on the most), and even how you define orgasm.

What are the Benefits of Orgasm?

There are dozens of benefits! Here is my selection of the 18 best health reasons to have orgasms.

- Increases cardio-vascular fitness
- Improves heart health
- Burns calories
- Improves skin (tone and quality)
- Builds and tones muscles
- Improves circulation
- Improves and maintains sexual function and health
- Improves and maintains the health of pelvic floor muscles
- Improves a woman's resistance to yeast infections
- Improves a man's resistance to prostate gland infections
- Lowers the risk of prostate cancer up to 60%
- Relieves some types of chronic pain
- Relieves symptoms of PMS
- Bolsters the adult auto-immune system
- Relieves stress
- Combats depression
- Reduces risk of endometriosis in women
- Reduces cortisol (which triggers fatigue)

To assure you that the data is there, here's a TINY sample of recent studies:

➡ a study at Rutgers University showed that sex improves problem-solving skills and teamwork

➡ a study at University of Paisley (Scotland) showed that sex reduces nervousness

➡ a study at Arizona State University showed that sex improves mood in women

➡ the *Journal of Epidemiology and Community Health* reported that orgasms 2 or more times per week reduces men's risk of a fatal heart attack by 50%

- a study at the New England Research Institute of Massachusetts, also showed that orgasms 2 or more times per week lowers the risk of heart disease

- a study at the National Cancer Institute showed that five or more orgasms (in men) per week significantly lowered the risk of prostate cancer

- the *British Journal of Urology International* reported that five or more orgasms per week reduces prostate cancer risk by a third in young men

- the *Journal of the American Medical Association* reported that 21 or more orgasms per month decreases the risk of prostate cancer in older men

- a study at Yale University showed that women who orgasm frequently reduce the risk of endometriosis

- the *Bulletin of Experimental Biology and Medicine* reported that oxytocin released during sex can reduce all forms of pain by up to 50%

- a study at Wilkes University, Pennsylvania showed that sex boosts the immune system

As I said, these are but a small fraction of the studies on sexual health in the last several years whose data conclude that orgasms promote improved human health and longevity.

Non-genitocentric Orgasm

When most people want an orgasm, they go straight to their genitals. Most but not all: sexual pleasure and orgasm may also be triggered by stimulation to non-genital areas anywhere on the body. Though considerably less common than people who react best to genital touching, there is considerable anecdotal data on people who climax when you deliver sensations to places on their body you might never before have considered sexual. We do not yet have an explanation for why this is: we only know that it is. I've heard hundreds of stories from adults who can achieve climax without direct genital stimulation.

Perhaps the most common non-genitocentric orgasm is the nipple orgasm. Depending on the natural level of sensitivity in your nipples, you may be able to give yourself an orgasm just by rubbing and stimulating your nipples. Generally speaking, female nipples are more sensitive than men's, but, as always, variations are the norm. There are volumes of anecdotal evidence that men not only deeply enjoy nipple stimulation but can climax from it, whether it's light touching or sucking or intense pinches and clamping.

Similarly kinky people, BDSMers, and fetishists may climax from a spanking, bondage, or a whipping. Some people can climax from giving — not receiving — sensation, particularly when they do so orally. I've spoken with men and women over the years who have been so aroused performing oral sex or analinctus that they climaxed from the psychological thrill of performing so intimate an act. Finally, all men have the potential for ejaculation through gentle massage of their prostate gland.

I think non-genitocentric orgasms break down into four camps:

➤ Being biologically predisposed to have special sensitivity in a non-erogenous zone. I've spoken to many men, for example, who are more quickly aroused by kisses and soft lipping of their ears than by direct touch to their penis. "Partialism" is a sub-category of fetishism which describes people who have a fetish for parts of the body (as opposed to objects like rubber or shoes). I worked with a partialist who preferred rubbing his feet to his genitals as foreplay, and only moved his hand back to his penis when he was ready to ejaculate.

➤ Environment or nurturing that make non-genital areas seem sexier. Some people grow up with such pleasant associations of body parts — like hands, hair or feet — that they can have orgasms from caressing or kissing them. Though rare, there are some people who grow up with such profound inhibitions that they redirect their desires away from their genitals because they can't bear the shame of touching them and essentially retrain themselves to eroticize less sexually threatening parts of the body.

● Learning by necessity to receive pleasure through non-genital-focused stimulation. I've worked with paralyzed clients who compensated for their inability to self-stimulate with their hands by eroticizing other acts, other body parts or by learning to receive a higher level of pleasure from the kind of light stimulation they may derive from clothing or undergarments rubbing against them. I once spoke with a quadriplegic man who had found a way to rub himself against the wrinkles in his adult diapers and bring himself to orgasm that way.

● Deliberate self-improvement. For the "gourmets" of masturbation, discovering new paths to orgasm is an art and a discipline. Tantric and other esoteric or pagan spiritual movements have long embraced full-body awareness and whole-body orgasms. They approach sexuality as a spiritual practice and invest time and effort to expand their boundaries. Masturbation techniques may be as esoteric as using your mind, breathing, or holding a position to create an orgasmic experience.

Transgender Orgasm

With the evolution of sex and gender roles in the 21st century, transgender issues must be included. As I am not a true expert in this area, I will keep my comments brief.

The great challenge for me, as a therapist, is that as varied as sexuality already is, transgendered people (whether they are cross-dressers, intersexed or something else) can be so individualistic in their sexual identity that I seldom meet two TGs with the same exact issues. A review of the literature assures me this is true even for therapists who specialize in transgenderism. Suffice to say that orgasm may be problematic for a transgendered person from birth to post-op; or it may never be a problem at all.

In my experience, most cross-dressers are no more or less likely than anyone else to be completely sexually functional. However, conflict or confusion over gender identity may lead to stress which then interferes with sexual urges.

For others, those stresses may begin at birth. For example, those born believing they have the "wrong genitals" may hate to touch them. Their genitals may feel alien and strange, and their capacity to experience pleasure through them varies, again depending on the individual. I worked with a 30-something transwoman who had never had partnered sex: she was waiting until corrective surgery gave her the "right genitals."

Physicians are able to construct a realistic vagina and retain orgasmic capability by using the penis to create a clitoris, so post-op women (transwomen) look and sexually respond more or less as biological women. The more or less depends on the skill of the surgeon and the candidate's own biology (successful recovery, good libido, stable hormone levels). Obviously, attitude plays a big role, and so do expectations: post-operative transwomen report orgasms that range from wildly exciting to very disappointing, with most post-op trans falling somewhere in the middle range and experiencing some diminishment in pleasure as compared with their pre-op responses. Complicating our ability to assess all of this accurately is the fact that orgasm is such a subjective and varied experience in the first place that we can only rely on how people describe their feelings about it.

It is not possible to construct a naturally functioning penis, or to give post-op transmen the ability to climax with their new equipment. Many female-to-male transsexuals opt to leave their female reproductive system intact, and thus continue to have orgasms and sexual pleasure with their biological genitals.

Orgasmic Dysfunctions

The inability to get aroused or to remain aroused during a sexual experience always has an underlying cause. The challenge is accurately diagnosing the cause. Here is a quick summary of common types of orgasmic dysfunction and the types of treatments that can correct them.

No Libido/No Arousal:

Complete lack of a libido is not normal and indicates an underlying health condition or a psychological issue.

We hold the odd cultural belief that a low sex drive is a good thing and lack of a sex drive sometimes best of all. We also seem to believe that women who claim they never feel in the mood, or who "just don't like sex that much" are perfectly normal. To me, these are tragic delusions. The truth is the opposite: a robust sex drive is a sign of good health and the absence of sex drive is a sign of deep trouble. The Latin phrase "health body, healthy mind" should include "healthy sexuality," because sex drive is critical to human identity.

As a rule of thumb, if you do not feel like having an orgasm at least two or three times a month (and more than that in your 20s and 30s) something is likely interfering with your natural biological needs. Your first stop should be a medical doctor. Specialists such as gynecologists, urologists, and endocrinologists are all equipped to check hormone levels, the usual culprit in sex drive disorders. If the problem isn't physical, then it is probably emotional: either something going on in one's life right now is repressing one's sexual energies, or some past trauma has left its wound in the form of a permanent shadow over one's ability to feel sexually alive.

Some medical conditions and their treatments deal a heavy blow to libido which, unfortunately, cannot be rectified. Women who have had double oophorectomies (removal of both ovaries) are at the highest risk of losing their appetite for sex. Old age can also dry up our needs for sex. But a reasonably healthy person should, in my opinion, make it a goal to maintain sexual activity as long as physically possible.

Some of us become asexual for emotional reasons, but people born asexual are rare. Many people who identify as asexual may well have undiagnosed sexual problems of either a physical or emotional nature.

Erectile Dysfunction:

My clinical view is that there are two types of ED: chronic and situational. The most common ED is situational — a passing failure that can be connected to a life event (losing a game, drinking too much, having an argument). Quite a few men have experienced ED when they are sleeping with someone who doesn't turn them on or they don't feel comfortable with. Although you may not admit it out loud, if you are with the wrong partner, your penis may speak for you. Situational ED is a normal event in the course of a man's life — sooner or later it happens to almost every man at least once, and typically more times than that. It is seldom a problem unless the man becomes so worried about it, he worries himself into chronic ED.

Chronic ED is a repeated inability to raise and maintain an erection to orgasm, whether alone or with a partner. Men over 60 are most vulnerable, as age takes its toll on the reproductive system, but ED may begin at any decade of adult life. According to recent studies, the majority of cases of chronic ED have a physiological cause (although some men develop chronic ED as a result of severe emotional conflicts). There are sophisticated medical treatments and drugs available now, with an impressive rate of success. However, there are no guarantees, particularly if the ED is associated with a major illness. So while a majority of patients may regain full erectile function with proper treatment, some cases resist treatment, or can only be resolved if and when the underlying organic issue is resolved.

Some men must adjust to life without full erections, just as some women must adjust to life without a full libido (after certain reproductive surgeries). It most certainly can be done. I firmly believe that if one discards the RM model as the ideal, one can continue to enjoy a rewarding and satisfying sex life even after a permanent physical change in sex drive and capabilities. I discuss new models of male and female sexuality in upcoming volumes.

ED is either organic (symptomatic of a medical problem) or psychological. One may, of course, lead to the other (a person can stress out so much, they make themselves sick; or what began as a medical condition may negatively impact moods and magnify stress). I use a quick and dirty technique to discern organic ED from a typical case of failing to perform in bed with a partner: I ask if he can masturbate to orgasm. If a man can maintain an erection during masturbation and achieve climax, he does not have an underlying organic issue. Everything is working fine, physically. The problem is an emotional issue which manifests during sex with a partner.

The range of emotional causes behind ED include low self-esteem, sexual shame, a sexual identity disorder, insecurity, performance anxiety, inhibition, fear of commitment, fear of intimacy, and poor body image or body dysmorphia (a hatred of your own body). I always ask clients to describe their lives so I can better understand the stresses they are dealing with, whether it's confusion about a relationship or the loss of a job. Sometimes, the problem turns out to be the partner: a bad sex partner can be worse than no partner at all and can transform the quality of one's sexual performance from good to awful. I've "cured" several men of situational ED by pointing out that their impotence was situational, thus reassuring them they were not on the slippery slope to permanent impotence — a fear which can devolve into a self-fulfilling prophecy.

Many of the drugs and medications prescribed for medical conditions (mood disorders, depression, diabetes, high blood pressure) can have a direct impact on the penis' ability to perform. Men who cannot maintain erections or climax from masturbation, but who are not on drugs, should get a medical exam to determine the cause, as organic ED can be indicative of underlying health problems, including heart disease. Obesity has been repeatedly proven to be a cause of diminished function, as the extra weight impinges on circulation to the pelvic region.

Premature Orgasm:

Culturally and medically, premature *ejaculation* (in men) is treated as a dysfunction (which it may or may not be, depending on the individual), and have ignored the fact that women too have ill-timed orgasms. I blame this on our creaky patriarchal culture's emphasis on the importance of the penis in coupled sex. Women too may have a premature climax, i.e., a very quick, disappointing or barely noticeable orgasm. We just haven't studied the female phenomenon nor accepted that female performance is as critical to a good sex life as male performance. An involuntary orgasm in a much shorter time-frame than expected or hoped occurs in both sexes, and I think we should call the phenomenon "premature orgasm" and find solutions for both men and women.

Research has shown that premature ejaculation in men has a genetic link: men who have PE are often the sons of men who have PE. If we can, one day, establish the full aetiology, physicians may find a cure for it. Thus far, most of the treatment for PE has been behavioral. For example, sexologists encourage men or women who feel they climax "too soon" to spend more time masturbating, and learning techniques to gain more control over their own responses.

Techniques include "taking the edge off" with an initial orgasm, and giving yourself enough recovery time to feel lustful again but not as anxious as the first time. More effective is to practice masturbation purposefully — taking breaks to extend the period of arousal; distracting yourself with non-sexual thoughts when you start to feel yourself beginning to orgasm; stopping all sexual stimulation and doing something else for a few minutes before resuming; and even clamping down on or pinching the genitals both to force back the blood flow and add a disagreeable sensation to delay or discourage orgasm. (Of course, if clamping down only adds to the excitement, a different kind of sensation should take its place.)

Slow to Orgasm:

Though it's not a common complaint, I know anecdotally that many people out there find it takes much longer than they (or their partners) wish for them to achieve climax. The reason that it isn't a common complaint is because, for some people, it's actually a plus. They may enjoy being able to spend more time on sensuality and arousal; and their partners may appreciate their ability to keep going and going while making love.

Still, some people find it frustrating, particularly if they or their partner experience discomfort in the process. These discomforts include feeling vasoconstriction in the genital region (which may express itself as pain), abrasion in the delicate genital tissues of the penis or vagina from long periods of rubbing or thrusting (particularly if you do not use an artificial lubricant), fatigue, back, muscle or joint pain from repetitive motion stress, and more.

The causes of slowness are many: from underlying emotional issues, to individual genetic disposition, aging, and degree of excitement. There are no drugs as yet to speed things up, though there are hundreds of sex tips in books and magazines to improve arousal by adding "spice" to your sex life. This may include new sexual positions, new and different types of stimulation, acting out sexual fantasies, and other creative ways to pump up your sexual chemistry and speed up your orgasmic response.

Lack of Orgasm:

Perhaps one of the most common problems sexologists treat, most especially with female clients, is the inability to climax, or inorgasmia.

In men, it's been my clinical experience that if they can maintain full erections, they can usually climax. Lack of climax in men seems to go along with ED (although even men who cannot achieve a full erection can have orgasms).

Inability to orgasm is a common female complaint. Its most common cause is the fluctuation in hormone levels women experience throughout their lives. As women grow into adulthood, their libido may rise or fall before and during menstruation, during ovulation, during and after pregnancy, before, during and after menopause, or as a result of reproductive surgeries and medications (particularly anti-depressants). Although somewhat rare, the side effects of birth control pills may include decreased sex drive and diminished orgasmic function in women. In extreme cases, birth control pills may permanently impair female function.

While hormones play an inestimably critical role in women's sex lives, the cultural and emotional baggage of being raised female in our culture have an enormous impact on female sex drive and ability to climax. Many female complaints mandate a trip to the doctor. In my experience, the roots of inorgasmia are usually emotional and should be treated with therapy.

How to Be a Sex Addict

Before moving on to the next section, an in-depth guide to healthier models for male and female sexuality, I'd like to offer a contemporary and science-based analysis of the difference between someone who likes sex a lot and someone who one might call a "sex addict."

Although we are no longer prey to Victorian quackery, new generations of quacks have taken their place. The pervasive belief that sexual behaviors which fall outside of the RM are diseases which require a cure has been a cash bonanza for hustlers and charlatans of every stripe. To me, the nadir of modern society's ignorance about sexuality is embodied by the Sex Addiction movement's fundamentally anti-sex philosophy. Thousands of people with healthy libidos are being hoodwinked into believing there's something wrong with them. Millions more believe that anyone who looks at porn or jerks off is a sex addict and needs treatment.

In fact, "sex addiction" is not a legitimate medical diagnosis: it is not listed in the DSM (Diagnostics and Statistic Manual), the diagnostic bible of mental illness and pathology. The term was coined by a doctor who built his practice by treating the condition he himself named. That so many people have since jumped on the Sex Addiction wagon is to me less a statement about sexual behavior than it is about our culture's fears and inhibitions about sex.

We continue to believe that there is such a thing as "too much sex," as if sex itself was a problem. I don't think sex is a problem. I think the problem is that people make lousy choices. All the time. Whether it's a president who selfishly chose a moment's pleasure over his responsibility to the nation he led, a revered athlete who is revealed to be a two-timing creep, or an actor who has gone on a binge of sex and drugs, the real cause of their bad sexual behaviors is an inability to make the right moral choices. In my clinical experience, I've also observed that people who make poor moral choices about sex tend to make poor moral choices in other areas as well. Also, as mentioned earlier, the people most likely to make self-destructive or self-sabotaging sexual choices are usually struggling with profound emotional conflicts about sex. Their internal confusion may influence a spectrum of social behaviors, including the ability to distinguish truth from lies or a feeling that the normal rules of life do not apply to them.

Currently, people who are trying to sell the American public on the idea of a "cure" for sexual addiction are liberally diagnosing as many people as possible. Although his theories of addiction have been debated and dismissed as quackery by the psychiatric establishment, Dr. Patrick Carnes — a chief architect of the Sex Addiction movement — exerts a huge influence over the diagnosis and treatment of sex addition. In his guide to "behaviors associated with sexual addiction," he includes masturbation, consistent use of pornography, unsafe sex, voyeurism, and phone sex as indicative of addiction. In this same diagnostic tool (which he encourages readers to use to assess themselves), he also lists sexual harassment and rape as symptoms of addiction. In other words, anyone who either enjoys non-RM sex or, on the other hand, commits sexual violence are equal members of the vast sex addiction club and require treatment by sex addiction specialists.

Not only are these ideas insulting, they are, in my view, a lame repackaging of Victorian ideology. The basis for this broadly generic diagnosis of "sexual addiction" is the assumption that the ideal sexual behavior for adults is to be monogamous with their partners, celibate when single, to repress sexual fantasies, not to think about sex too frequently, and not to be interested in sexual variety or new sexual experiences. Perhaps the most irritating aspect of the sexual addiction folly is that it is predicated on the notion that sex is fundamentally bad. Therefore the more you think about sex, the more you engage in it, and the less you focus on reproductive sex with a monogamous partner, the "sicker" you are.

Sex can be addictive, of course. Anything that makes a person feel good and helps them escape from daily problems can be addictive. We don't treat rabid sports fans as addicts, but they are. They crave the highs of victory and wrap themselves in the glory of the game, sometimes to the detriment of real people or events in their lives. We shake our heads at shopaholics, and feel sorry for people who struggle with food addictions. We don't stigmatize them as perverts. Anyone who feels a visceral hunger and emptiness inside may try to fill that void, whether it's with gambling, Gucci purses or sex. The pleasures of the moment smooth all of life's rough edges — until the moment ends, of course.

In the 21st century, the scientific understanding of sexuality is that genuine sexual disorders are symptomatic of other disorders, either medical or psychological. Treatment for the underlying disorder is the first step towards improved sexual health. I've never met a self-described or previously diagnosed sex addict who was actually addicted to sex per se: they usually had low self-esteem, poor impulse control, obsessive/compulsive disorders and more than a few had underlying personality disorders that undermined their ability to make good choices overall. Only occasionally do I meet someone who I would consider really hooked on sex. Even then, treatment still begins by trying to understand the drivers.

A sex addiction should stand up to the same criteria as other addictions:

➤ *Your sexual impulses and behaviors interfere with your daily life — work, friends, family suffer because you place your sexual needs above all else.* Examples: spending the rent money on sexual pleasures, avoiding intimacy with a partner or failing to provide your children with quality time, missing or screwing up at work because you can't stop thinking about sex — all of these suggest you are using sex to avoid real world responsibilities. People with a history of substance addiction are particularly at risk; even after they get sober, they may act out all the same dysfunctional and self-destructively addictive behaviors in their sex lives.

➤ *You cannot control when, where, how or with whom you have sex.* Examples: thinking any opportunity for sex is a good one, even when you know consciously that it isn't; consistently giving in to pressure from others and being unable to say no; consistently engaging in acts or behaviors that you know are bad for your health; giving into spontaneous urges, even when they mean taking dangerous risks with your health, reputation or fortune.

In other words, a sexual addiction should mean that you are completely out of control of your "habit," just like the junkie or drunk who is out of control. Using porn, talking or visiting sex-workers, frequent masturbation are all perfectly acceptable choices for adults as long as they are able to function normally in the world and make health-positive choices about the who/how/when/where of partnered sex.

The inclusion of rapists on the same list as people who masturbate and watch Internet porn is deeply troubling to me. That's like putting an axe-murderer on the same list as the elderly aunt who pinches your cheeks a little too hard. Nor does the list make the critical distinction between "chronic" and "situational." There are times in an adult's life when he or she may over-indulge in sex or otherwise make bad sexual choices. To anyone seriously committed to helping the patient, it is absolutely critical to know if such behavior is situational (happening in response to a stressful life-event, for example) or an ingrained and long-term pattern of behavior. Treatment must vary accordingly or you end up causing more harm than good.

Far from being a bad thing, as the Sex Addiction Movement implies, it's important for adults to masturbate and find other safe sources of sexual satisfaction, particularly when they don't have a partner around. Sexual variety is natural and normal, and helps keep one sexually vibrant. Many couples share a healthy interest in sex toys, online hot-chat, masturbation, voyeurism, exhibitionism, fetishism, and more of the behaviors the Sex Addiction Movement considers symptomatic of addiction.

By the addiction standards set by Carnes, every man and women who works in the sex industry (from professional call girls and strippers to the millions of ladies who upload amateur photos to the Internet, to movie directors, adult toy store owners, and porn actors) is a sex addict. When millions of people can so easily qualify for a diagnosis, it's a good guess something is wrong with the diagnosis and not the people.

Section Two

THINKING ABOUT SEX

ᕙ Introduction ᕗ

---◦---

This section is devoted to ideas and understandings I implement in my therapy practice. Some of the concepts are widely known and debated in sex-related fields. Some are working theories I've developed independently and am writing about for the first time. Combined, they aim to form a contemporary, fact-based framework for an adult understanding of sex and its role in daily life.

For example, the intrinsic connections between mind and body, long considered a matter of Eastern religious theory, has been researched and affirmed by western science. This holistic view must now be factored into a healthy life, and with it, an awareness of the unbreakable bond between personal identity and sexual identity.

The role of talking as a means of healing from sexual damages is another important concept, particularly in a culture which generally shuts down "embarrassing" conversation about sex. For, while the link between language skills and cognition is a widely accepted fact, and though we know that an inability to articulate experience usually correlates with an inability to learn from that experience, no one has yet stated the obvious: you need to be able to talk about sex in order to be able to think about sex rationally. Without a language for sex, adults do not mature sexually. They become trapped in adolescent cycles, feeling and acting much as they did in their teens, typically defining sex at age 50 the way they defined it at age 20.

I also offer some of my own ideas about the best reasons to have sex, along with a long section on "Sexual Intelligence" and its importance in adult sexuality. Along the way, I delve into the biology of sex and the role of free will in human sexual behavior. While I am a great believer in candid advice and sexual techniques, the upcoming concepts and perspectives are, in fact, what most transform my clients' lives.

↜ Chapter Four ↠

Talking About Sex

———◈———

Talking = Thinking = Healing

The single biggest obstacle to greater levels of sexual health and well-being among adults is the absence of open, calm, and sensitive public discussion of sexual issues in our society. If we can't talk about sex, then it is impossible to think critically about sex. And, if we can't think critically about sex, we cannot develop maturity or wisdom about the subject. For those reasons we remain, as a culture, adolescent in our sexual attitudes and behaviors, and intellectually mired in 19th century beliefs. Moreover, I believe it's why people are still so confused and mystified about sex; they don't know what they should know, and many of the things they think they know about sex are simply wrong.

Out-dated ideologies still control the debate about sex. Think of all the times one hears so-called experts on matters of love, marriage and sex espouse the same old notions:

- that the only moral sex is sex between married heterosexuals
- that infidelity means (or should mean) the end of a marriage
- that sexual variations are abnormal
- that men have a stronger sex drive than women
- that all women and all men naturally adhere to fixed standards of sexual normalcy

Myths like these are so frequently repeated, even by sex and relationship experts, that they form the backbone of contemporary public opinions about sex. And, again, they are all wrong, at least if we examine the wealth of evidence which has repeatedly proven them wrong.

Several years back, Gina G., a rather rich lady called me. She had listed me as number three on her call-list of famous sex therapists, and after consulting the first two was more confused than before. Both were far better known than me, regularly surfacing on radio and television shows, with reams of books to their credit. I doubted I could offer her better advice than they'd given. Until I heard her problems and the advice they'd given her. Suffice to say, better some people should sell fish rather than advise the profoundly troubled souls who occasionally show up in a sex therapist's practice.

On the surface, she was having difficulty achieving orgasms with her boyfriend during sex. But the story she told involved infinitely more than their current issues with sexual intercourse — their trust in each other was nil, their history of acrimony was frightening, they had a very unwholesome co-dependency, and both of them had deeply unhappy, dysfunctional personal histories. Yet, instead of helping Gina to accept that her issues went far, far beyond orgasms and would require a comprehensive treatment approach (therapy and medication), they both gave her technical tips on positions, exercises, and lubricants.

She faithfully followed their advice but it didn't work, as anyone with a solid education in the field would have predicted. By providing nothing more than some friendly advice on "try it this way" or "touch that place," they encouraged her in the common misbelief that sex is of the body and that if you can just find the right position or magic touch, your sex problems will be solved.

It is a common fantasy among people who are suffering that there is a magic bullet: a simple, easy, painless, solution that will put them out of a lifetime of misery in one easy step. It is a responsible helping professional's obligation to wake people up from that fantasy. Unfortunately, so many of our most famous experts do the opposite: in sound-bytes and blurbs, they encourage the consumer to believe that the solution is a one-size-fits-all proposition.

Needless to say I'm also irked that my colleagues encouraged Gina, already in denial about the scope of her problems, in the delusion that sex is purely of the body and can be solved purely through the body. One fact that all adults should and must know is that sex is as much of the mind as it is of the body. The belief that "if you do it the way everyone does it" or "if you move your pelvis this way instead of that way" will be enough to get someone past deep emotional hurts that are inhibiting them from embracing their sexual potential is not only naïveté, it's chicanery.

As I sometimes remind clients, if one layers years of problems on top of problems, you have to give yourself a generous cushion of time to heal before you are going to achieve your optimal potential. We all hear about the negative impact of stress on our bodies; we don't hear nearly enough about its impact on our minds. Every fight, every crisis, every rejection, every misunderstanding may inflict damage. Years of feeling profoundly conflicted about your sexuality creates cumulative damage.

It's disturbing to think about how much money adults spend on unnecessary surgeries, sex toys, and experts who are ill-equipped to delve into the critical mass of sexual identity. Although most of my clients blanch when they realize I am going to ask them a lot of questions — on topics as varied as childhood environment and relationships, their family structure and relations, details on when they began masturbating, their relationship history since adolescence, and their health status — every one of those questions may be material to their adult sexual patterns.

As numerous studies have shown, the best, most successful method for overcoming emotional obstacles and damages is talk therapy. While medication (such as anti-depressants) provide an indispensable function in stabilizing moods and emotions so one may calmly deal with issues, it is only by actually dealing with those issues and by talking about them, that healing occurs.

Scientific studies have demonstrated that bottled up stress alters the brain for the worse; they have similarly shown that the relief of talking alters the brain for the better and actually heals the brain of stress-related damage. Since sex is as much of the brain as the body, your sexual appetites, choices, and performance are distorted by stress. The way you think about sex, and about your own sexuality, change. Depression or chronic health issues compound the problem.

Yet, I've seen miraculous transformations in even the most difficult, self-described "hopeless cases." It's slow work at times. It can take years. But by learning to articulate thoughts, and apply critical skills to their sexual choices, I've seen client after client discover sexual potentials within themselves they didn't know they had. The work is all based on good counseling practice but sometimes the results feel magical.

When Talk is the Best Medicine

Kevin T. was a 45-year-old professional athlete, tall, handsome, and usually very affable. But lately, he was sunk in gloom. For the first time in his life, he was having ED. It had shaken him to the core. He couldn't accept that it was happening to him; at the same time, he was obsessed with the fear that his gorgeous, long-time girlfriend would leave him if he couldn't satisfy her.

He went to his doctor, who sent him to specialists who discovered his testosterone was on the low end. They began the standard treatment and he kept waiting for something to change. Six months later, nothing had changed. He kept hoping to feel that familiar old surge of enthusiasm in his pants when they kissed but it wasn't happening. He decided it would be best to avoid sex rather than risk another humiliating failure in bed. Now he was wondering if it was more than physical and wondered if a therapist could help him.

After a few questions, I learned that he had no difficulties masturbating to orgasm in private. Since the testosterone treatments, in fact, masturbation was feeling even better than before. Had an MD asked him the right questions, he would have known to refer my client to a sex therapist immediately. If a man can achieve erection and orgasm when masturbating, but cannot do the same when having partnered sex, the problem is not organic. The problem is psychological.

I was very glad that Kevin had his testosterone levels checked. In my perfect world of sexual medicine, every man would get a baseline testosterone screen around the same age women get their baseline mammograms. Since his numbers were on the low end, it was especially helpful, as his doctors would now be keeping an eye on those all-important androgen levels. The boost to his masturbatory function was a bonus. But did it warrant all the expensive tests, the topical gels, and the injections? He wasn't sure. What he did know was that he had spent a small fortune on doctors and treatments and he still couldn't make love to his girlfriend. Now he was wondering if anyone could cure him or if he had to resign himself to a lonely life without sex or a girlfriend. What became glaringly clear to me within a few sessions was that he was preoccupied with his own definitions of masculinity — in sum, "a man must always be hard at will or he is not a man" — and his assumptions that his girlfriend must now think of him either with pity or scorn because he couldn't get it up. He was so preoccupied that he was unable to step back and apply some common sense to what was really going on.

After competing in an exhausting race, he and his girlfriend joined a group at a local pub to celebrate. They ate steaks and drank wine. By the time they got home that night, they were both exhausted and cranky. They argued over something inconsequential, then decided to have make-up sex. Except they didn't because he could not get an erection. Tired and embarrassed, they both just rolled over and went to sleep. They didn't talk about it the next day. Or ever again. After two weeks of this, it became the elephant in the room, and after a month without sex, they both exploded one night and had a very ugly fight about the lack of sex. He went to his doctor that very week. Now, eight months later, he was sitting in my office.

What had begun as a moment's failure after a long night of partying to celebrate a big win had spiraled into a mania of anxiety, frustration and self-doubt. He was one of those very rare and, as I see it, lucky men who had not experienced ED until his 45th year. Lucky because most men have at least one or two episodes of ED before then. This was part of his problem: he was in denial about getting older. At 45, he could no longer lead the frat-boy lifestyle. If he played hard all day and drank all night, chances were that, at his age, he would be happier cozying up to a teddy bear than a horny woman when he finally hit the sack. His ED was the result of a combination of very common factors: pushing his body too hard, ignorance of the multitude of factors that can cause temporary ED, and a distorted perspective on masculinity which placed all the emphasis on his sex organs. If they didn't work, then he himself was "broken."

My treatment plan was deceptively simple. First on the agenda was taking better, more respectful care of his aging body. This included better food, less alcohol, and at least 7 hours of restful sleep every day. Second, whether or not he felt confident about his erections, I asked that he resume intimacy with his girlfriend as soon as possible. If he was worried she'd leave him for not being adequately stout, then chances were even better she'd leave him if he ignored her sexual needs completely. He hoped that by avoiding sex altogether he'd avoid dealing with their sexual problems, a common misconception. I cautioned him that the reverse was true: the more you avoid the problems, the more complicated, even overwhelming, they become. The most productive strategy was to take small steps in the right direction.

Instead of making their sex life all about his own ability to get it up, I suggested they focus on the other things they enjoyed together, such as oral sex and mutual massaging and caressing, and that he try to give her orgasms even when he wasn't going to have one. I was sympathetic to his anxiety about being naked with her again, but told him that if he really wanted to hang on to his woman, he had to treat her sexual needs as equal to his and at least help her to feel pleasure and relief through intimacy. In choosing to avoid sex, he was essentially putting her sex life on hold and raising the risk of her walking away in sexual frustration.

As we talked, he developed insights about his sexual attitudes. He worked on developing more rational expectations, and realized that his masculine identity had been too tied to one part of his body. In his head he knew better but until he talked it all out, he had not been able to shake his programming that — in effect — a man was only as good as his erections.

He learned about ED and was vastly relieved to find out that, in most cases, it's temporary. We talked about prevention strategies for right now, and preparation for the effects of aging in years to come. I assured him that if he continued to do the things he was doing now, he might well be able to remain sexually active until the end of his life. Perhaps what was most therapeutic of all was that he was able to unburden himself completely of his shame and anxiety with someone who did not think he was any less of a man for having this problem, and who could fill in all the gaps in his knowledge about how the male body and mind work together.

He was shocked at how quickly things turned around for him. His girlfriend was thrilled with the attention and affection she was getting from him. Non-penetrative intimacy with his girlfriend had made them more creative in bed. Thinking up new ways to give and receive pleasure brought an unanticipated bonus: it made them feel even closer than before. It helped free her up too, as she felt more comfortable telling him what she liked and how she liked it.

The less he worried about his performance, the better he took care of his sexual health, and the more ways he found of stimulating and pleasuring his girlfriend, the more he felt in charge of his masculinity. In a few weeks, he was back to his old self in bed. As he put it, "It's like someone flipped a switch." I considered it a genuine triumph for him that he decided to continue mixing things up in bed. He had thought it all through and realized that not only had it brought them closer as a couple but that it would be more relaxing to him to know he could give her pleasure even when they were old and their bodies not as sexually spry as in their prime.

Though his testosterone may medically be on the low end, and though he will need to be routinely screened to keep an eye on those numbers, Kevin's sex life is back where it was before that awful ED night and, according to him, even better than before because there's more variety.

Talking About the Truth

Over the years, any number of people made appointments with me not because of their sexual problems per se but because they hungered for non-judgmental dialogue about sex. For many clients, the simple ability to speak without inhibition is a profound relief. The more they talk about it, the more relaxed they feel about it. The more they know about the science of sex, the clearer their understanding of how it fits into their own lives. The more answers they get to their questions, the more they mature, the smarter they become, the richer and more complex their understanding of sex (and life, for that matter), and, ultimately, the better their choices in love and relationships.

One of the sweetest rewards of being a sex therapist is the incredible gratitude one receives from clients, as if one has conjured special powers to perform magic. Few of the people who come to me have genuine faith that their lives will change for the better. They have that hope and realize they must at least make the effort, but after growing up in a culture which sends so many ambiguous messages about sex, and all too many outright hateful stereotypes of sexual behaviors, they assume that there are no real answers for sexual problems.

But there are. Every day we are getting more information, and richer understandings, of sexual problems. A reawakening of the scientific study of sex is occurring in the 21st century. An awful lot has changed in the scientific understanding of sex since the 19th century, and most especially our understanding that sex is as much a matter of the brain as it is of the sex organs.

We know things Freud never dreamed. Today there is wide consensus among all sexologists that a realistic model of sexuality is nuanced and diverse, full of overlaps and gray areas. Masculine and feminine are not absolutely divided as previously believed: gender is fluid and variable. The boundaries between gay, bi and straight are blurrier than previously thought. Sexual responses are fantastically varied, in intensity and duration. Sexual appetites and preferences are as random and particularized as our food appetites and preferences.

A century ago, scientists routinely tried to treat sexual behaviors by addressing the symptoms, and measured normalcy against the reproductive standard. Today's sexologist doesn't accept that there must be one sexual standard for all people. He or she is more likely to focus on helping clients achieve their own potentials, and not strive to fit into a mold. To boil down everything we now know about human sexuality into one sound-byte: **diversity is normal.**

Yet somewhere down the line, between the 19th century when the study of sex was considered respectable and valuable to human progress — a time when sex scientists were lionized at home and abroad as geniuses who had unraveled some of life's greatest mysteries, their works widely read and debated — and the 20th century, the scientific dialogue about sex was hijacked by moralists and prudes.

There is an appalling information gap between what sex scholars know and what the public knows. The study of sexology itself remains too embarrassing and politically unpopular for most universities to support. Efforts to offer sex-positive education at high schools and universities invariably cause a public outcry. There are very few public platforms for research and opinions which go against the entrenched Victorian morality of American mores. Meanwhile, charlatans and unqualified talking heads continue to issue bad advice about sex and relationships, while quacks continue to sell penis enlargement pills and other fake remedies to an eternally gullible public. To say that this is frustrating to sexologists is an understatement. For those of us who are educated in the field, it's mind-bending to see people who are completely ignorant about sex making public policy about issues like STD control, sex education, and contraception.

The most compelling theory as to why sex has been cast into the gutter is that as long as scientists re-enforced ideas which upheld preconceived religious beliefs about sex, they were given a wide berth. When 20th century sex activists, scientists and thinkers issued data that conflicted with traditional morality, however, they were cast out from the public dialogue about sex and vilified for promoting corrupt and degenerate behaviors.

Respected 20th century researchers (Kinsey, Masters & Johnson, Bullogh) were issuing massive amounts of data showing that there was far more to normal, healthy human sexuality than the Reproductive Model (RM). Instead of the male-dominant, reproductive, pro-religion model, the emerging model of sexuality was more secular, more egalitarian, and placed a value on pleasure for women as well as men. Throughout 1920s US and Europe, increasing numbers of adults were exploring the possibilities: a proliferation of nudist/Naturist groups and movements emerged, as did many utopian free love communities, sacred sex societies, private fetish and bondage societies, gay and lesbian communities, and so on.

What was viewed as progress by sexually liberated individuals, however, incited a vicious backlash from those who staunchly defended the traditional patriarchal and religious structures of society. To political and religious conservatives, sex for pleasure was a selfish, sinful act, an abomination which threatened to destroy the very fabric of Judeo-Christian society. To suggest that adults could find an equal or greater sexual happiness outside of a church-sanctioned heterosexual marriage was denounced as a direct threat to morality.

By the time Alfred Kinsey published his ground-breaking study of adult sexuality in the late 1940's, conservative social forces were aligned against sexual enlightenment. Kinsey's work — arguably the first truly scientific, evidence-based, large-scale study of human sexuality — triggered a sex culture war that is still being fought today.

Kinsey, originally an entomologist who specialized in gall wasps, had observed that a range of variables (evolution, sex, class, age) caused differences in the insects' sexual behaviors. These data ultimately led Kinsey to consider whether scientific study of human sexuality would yield similar results. And so he began collecting and analyzing volumes of data which ultimately provided abundant evidence that sexual intimacy among adults does not operate on one fixed model but, instead, is variable. It's funny how obvious that is to us now, but in Kinsey's time, it was revolutionary to say that oral sex, masturbation, homosexuality, and bisexuality were within the spectrum of normal variations. Kinsey's work answered the questions that had been plaguing scientists since the 19th century, most pertinently why it was that so many of us didn't conform to the RM.

Unfortunately, very few people wanted to hear the answer Kinsey provided. Nor was it only moralists and prigs who rejected the science of sex. Long after Kinsey had amply demonstrated that sexual variations were common behaviors, not mental illnesses, the legal system clung to 19th century laws based on the unscientific theories and prejudices of the Victorians. Homosexuals, bisexuals, transgenderists, polyamorists, and all others who did not conform to the RM were — and in some places still are — subject to legal prosecution and prison at the whim of the courts.

Even more disappointing, the medical establishment resisted Kinsey's work. Psychiatrists continued to treat sexual variations as diseases and offered treatments, knowing full well they didn't work. For example, Kinsey was not the first to demonstrate that women freely enjoyed orgasmic sex and sexual variety. But until the late 1960s, female inorgasmia was considered normal by most doctors and men of science. Like their Victorian forebears, they generally believed that women didn't really enjoy sex or have an independent sex drive. Female sexual identity was shaped by duty to one's husband and country. Women who didn't want to have sex with their husbands were diagnosed as frigid, and treated with drugs and psychoanalysis to make them more submissive. Conversely, women who enjoyed frequent intercourse or multiple partners were diagnosed as nymphomaniacs and faced involuntary institutionalization, psychotropic drug treatments and worse to break them of their lustful ways.

And, while it may seem as if we've come a very long way from those dark middle-20th century ages, as a sex therapist, I'm all too painfully aware that, in fact, we have not.

Several years ago, Nina R. came to me because she was uncomfortable with the treatment plan prescribed by a psychiatrist and wanted a sex therapist's opinion on her problem. She was a happily married woman of 42, and for most of their 15-year marriage, she and her husband had enjoyed relations 7 to 10 times a week. For the past several months, however, he'd stopped initiating. They only made love now two or three times a week, and always at her request. Nina felt hurt, rejected, confused. He was never in the mood anymore. What did it mean?

The psychiatrist thought he knew: Ten times a week?! She was a nympho! She had worn her husband down to a hollow shell of a man with her insatiable lusts. Although he didn't officially diagnose her as a nymphomaniac (he couldn't, because it is no longer listed in the DSM) he said she had those tendencies and prescribed anti-depressants to balance her mind and blunt her sex drive. The psychiatrist didn't take a comprehensive history of the background details of the marriage. Instead, he wrote the prescription based on how many times he believed a couple should have sex — a belief which, of course, had nothing to do with science or facts. It isn't common for people to have sex every day but, as most sexologists know, the world would be a healthier place if they did. As far as I was concerned, Nina and her husband were to be congratulated for finding so much joy and intimacy in their marriage. Isn't that the point?

When I took her history, Nina mentioned that her husband had lost a well-paying job and didn't feel confident he would find another that paid half as well. I probed and discovered that he was so down about it, he barely left the house. He moped around, watching TV or playing games, and medicating his misery with beer and junk food. Not surprisingly, their sex life declined within weeks of this turn-around in his fortunes. The more she told me, the more I was appalled by the psychiatrist's treatment. If anyone needed anti-depressants, it was the husband. (Although, after seeing that psychiatrist, Nina really could have used something to soothe her nerves.)

I pointed out the obvious: a significant decline in her husband's sex drive right around the time he lost his job probably meant that his lack of desire for her was a symptom of his overall depression. Add alcohol to the mix, and it was a recipe for sexual dysfunction. My advice to her was that before she worked on the sex problems, she needed to help him get back on track, and push him to make healthier choices. As long as depression clouded his judgment, it would likely also continue to dampen his sex drive.

Her relief was palpable. She'd been so hurt by her husband's rejection, she couldn't step back and see the bigger picture. When the doctor told her she was too sexually demanding, she was embarrassed and ashamed. Were those 15 years of sexual bliss that they shared a hollow sham? Now she realized their problem was more likely a temporary setback. We discussed some things she could do to help affirm him and comfort him through his crisis and she left feeling optimistic.

I only saw her once. Nina wrote me a month later, expressing the deepest of gratitude. In a few short weeks, she'd gotten her husband to see a counselor and cut back on beer. They were going for long nightly walks, she was cooking more, and more nutritious, meals, and he was coming out of his shell. Their sex life was almost back to where it was before he got fired and the future looked bright.

She wasn't the first client who received a bad diagnosis for a sexual problem from a psychiatrist who was quick to judge a sexual behavior, rather than look at sex as a product of a complex set of forces, variations and circumstances.

I'll never forget the client who drove six hours to see me after a dissatisfying session with the most highly-recommended psychiatrist in his own state. He had consulted the psychiatrist about how his fetish had led to some reckless behavior, and the psychiatrist's advice boiled down to one sentence: "Don't think about it and it'll go away."

I have no idea what that psychiatrist actually knew about sex but clearly he was not keeping up with the literature. Fetishes do not go away. Not thinking about sex is not a cure for sex. Poor choices do not suddenly become good choices if you don't address the underlying issues and find a balance in yourself between what you want and what you may have.

Like the doctor who saw a woman who wanted sex every day as a disgusting nympho, I believe this psychiatrist was personally revolted by my client's (admittedly unusual) fetish. Perhaps it was the psychiatrist who didn't want to think about the fetish.

My client, however, had no choice, as a fetish is a permanent fixture of a person's sexual identity. He didn't believe that something he had been fantasizing about since childhood would just go away if he distracted himself with yard work or took up knitting. Neither did I.

In our work together, I advised him to accept that his fetish would likely always be with him. The fetish itself was sensual and harmless but his behaviors were self-destructive. Shame and desperation about the fetish had led him to spend money he didn't have and to go places he should have avoided. So we focused on improving his self-esteem, learning to accept his sexual quirks, and making sane, positive choices about how to conduct his sex life, now and in the future. I assured him that while a fetish does mean his dating pool is smaller, it did not by any means ruin his chances of finding a life-partner. Not only was there someone out there who had the same exact fetish, but he might also bump into a number of potential life-mates who didn't share the fetish but would be more than happy to explore it with him and would love him exactly as he was. Knowing that people with fetishes can lead full, healthy romantic and family lives, and that his pool of potential partners was larger than the people he randomly met in hidden Internet chat-rooms comforted him enormously.

A few facts about the realities of sex, and the relationship between overall behavior and sexual behavior, can make all the difference in the lives of some clients. In 2011, both frigidity and nymphomania have long-since been scrubbed from the DSM. Instead of nymphomania, there is now a diagnosis of hypersexuality applied to women who compulsively engage in sex and cannot feel fulfilled no matter how many times they have sex or how many partners they have with. But hypersexuality is no longer broadly applied to women simply because they enjoy having a lot of sex. Instead, there must be a medical basis for the diagnosis.

Similarly, today we recognize that the desire for vaginal intercourse isn't the unique standard by which one may judge a happy sex life. We know that some people are born with intensely high libidos and some with naturally low ones. We know some people feel "all girl" or "all boy" and others feel somewhere in between or something else that cannot be defined as uniquely male or female. We know that fetishes, sexual obsessions, quirks, weird fantasies, and all the other so-called abnormal or perverted behaviors are not indicative of criminal or unstable personalities but are, in fact, normal and fairly common features of human sexuality.

Variation, variability, diversity: those are the truths that set many of my clients free of false expectations and help them to embrace their individual sexual identity. If there is just one lesson I want all my clients to learn from therapy with me, it's that they should never let anyone make them feel guilty or flawed if their sexuality doesn't conform to a standard that was false in the first place.

⇥ Chapter Five ⇤

Defining Sex

———◄◦►———

How Do You Define Sex?

Just as I was getting down to writing this section, the Kinsey Institute issued what I consider to be one of the most important sex studies every conducted.

Kinsey researchers just proved that no one really knows how to define what is and is not sex. I was so happy to see it. I've been telling clients for years that no one knows, in hopes of assuring those whose sexuality was so far off the mainstream model that they felt hopelessly alone. I think I've known that no one knew what sex was since I was a teenager. As a wild hippie child, I considered accumulating sexual experiences to be a must-do project of adult life. It became quickly obvious that the hand-job that one boy considered a complete and even guilty sexual experience was what another boy considered a barely-acceptable consolation prize for lack of penetration. Now I finally have data to support what I always suspected: people define sex subjectively. There is no universal consensus on what sex really is.

The Kinsey study asked people if they considered oral sex to be sex, or only vaginal penetration to be sex, and how did they feel about masturbation — was that sex? In the end, results were all over the map. While 95% of the people surveyed believed sexual intercourse was sex, for example, some of them made exceptions depending on the circumstances of the intercourse. When it came to sex acts such as anal and oral sex, there was considerable disagreement on whether those acts were really sex or not.

Too bad the study wasn't around when President Clinton tried to explain that he didn't consider oral sex to be sex. People laughed or thought he was lying, but I knew he probably was genuinely confused. And why wouldn't he be? Several urban studies of high school students have shown that teenage girls don't equate oral sex with "real" sex and are willing to give their male friends blow-jobs on that basis. Personally, I always considered it a sexual event when a penis was in my mouth but in Kentucky, I'd be in the minority. A 2007 study of about 500 college students by the University of Kentucky showed that only one fifth (20%) of them thought that oral sex counts as sex, while 22% didn't believe that anal intercourse was sex either.

I think people should look at sex the way sexologists do. All sex-related behavior is sex. When you stimulate yourself with your hand, when you look at naughty pictures, when you flirt, when you have a fantasy, go to a strip club, go to a BDSM educational event, when you rush to the bookstore to get your favorite star to sign their new tell-all because you can't wait to read about their private love lives, it's all sexual, and mostly harmless. The problems arise when people disagree on how to define what is acceptable in their lives and relationships. Consider the parents who assume their daughter understands that "no sex before 18" means no sex before 18, while she, like her friends, thinks they only mean intercourse; or the life-partners who live side by side as sexual strangers to one another.

Defining Your Sexual Language

When couples come to me and say, "We want a better sex life," one of my first assignments to them is to sit down and define, as precisely as possible, what each one means by a better sex life. What's important to them — frequency? creativity? intensity? steel fetters and five inch heels? The details are germane.

Some people miss out on wonderful sexual opportunities because they assume their partner will share their own definitions. Bob and Renee F. had been happily married for several years but Bob called me, fearful that his interest in porn was tearing them apart. He defined porn as bad, and a type of cheating. He hated himself for sneaking onto X-rated sites, a teenage habit he thought would end when he got married. But the fact was the sites revved him up and made sex with his wife even hotter. Now things were falling apart because of his disgusting habit. When she peeked over his shoulder one night and joked about an image on the screen, he slammed his laptop shut and went ballistic. His over-reaction upset his wife: the more upset she got, the more distraught and guilty he felt.

He blamed the porn; I blamed his belief that porn was bad and that he had defined himself and his needs into a very cruel corner. Every time he gave in to what was, fundamentally, a harmless and normal urge, he loathed himself all the more. The worse he felt about himself the more he escaped into porn. To break that vicious cycle, he needed to examine his own attitudes towards sex. Was it realistic to expect a sexually healthy, virile man to never look at or think about another woman? Did his wife expect that of him? He described Renee as hip, progressive, and very open-minded. Perhaps if he had smiled at his wife's joke, or used it as an opportunity to open up about his sexual fantasies, things would have gone very differently.

When I met Renee, she looked like she was expecting a piano to fall on her head. She thought Bob was bringing her to a therapist to make a horrible, life-shattering confession. When we finally explained that Bob was struggling with his interest in porn, Renee's jaw dropped. This was about porn? She was incredulous. She knew he liked porn. She assumed most men did. She'd thought he was having an affair!

After her shock faded, Renee felt bad for Bob. She told him she wished they'd discussed it years ago. As far as she was concerned, it was okay if he looked at naked boobies, as long as the only ones he ever touched were hers. To Renee, the definition of cheating was strictly physical. When Bob heard that Renee defined porn as "stuff to fuel fantasies you act out with your partner" and monogamy as "physically faithful," a weight was lifted off his shoulders. Ironically, as Bob's guilt over looking at porn waned, his interest in it waned as well. He was able to put it into better perspective in his life and focus more energy on his well-deserving wife.

Warren J. was a sadder story. He came for support and counseling after his wife announced she wanted a divorce "out of the blue." He told me he was a great provider, he never cheated on her, he didn't smoke or drink. When he found out there was another man in the picture, he blamed the man for being a predator who had manipulated his wife.

The more I probed, though, the more I understood why his wife left. At home, he routinely locked himself in his office immediately after dinner, instructing her not to disturb his work. He did the same on weekends. As it turned out, he spent most of those hours surfing porn. As he defined it, porn wasn't really sex, so technically he wasn't cheating. He rationalized that porn helped him stay physically faithful. He didn't know what his wife did for sexual satisfaction. He assumed she didn't have much of a sex drive, another rationalization for looking at porn. His wife had asked him to see a marriage counselor with her a few months before the divorce, but he refused. He was afraid his porn habits would be exposed. So he closed his eyes to the situation and kept spending more time with his computer than with his wife.

Although Warren said he believed in monogamy, fidelity, true love, and marriage, his behavior did not support his own definitions. He behaved like a horny bachelor living with a roommate whose needs didn't really concern him. Warren's moral compass had drowned in a sea of sexual fluids. He showed many of the characteristics of an addict: excuses, lies, rationalizations, delusions, and selfishness. The consequence was predictable: his wife found someone who gave her the love she had been missing.

There would be no quick resolutions or happy outcomes for him until he either changed his definitions or changed himself. If he wanted a happier life, he had to learn how to get whatever it was that he needed from real life and stop using porn as a crutch. The next time he promised someone monogamy and love, he needed to be sure he knew what he meant when he used the words and he needed to understand what his partner meant. Otherwise, he would screw up his next marriage in all the same ways.

Sometimes, serious differences in how two people define sex and monogamy results in bizarre situations. My client Liz R. firmly believed that the missionary position sex was the only legitimate sex act between a man and woman. Her husband Lyle had bugged her to perform oral sex on him, but she thought it was degrading. She continued to maintain that oral sex wasn't real sex until Lyle confessed to getting a blowjob while away on business. At that point, Lucy had to face the fact that, actually, she did consider oral sex to be sex. She was jealous, heartbroken, enraged, and everything else one would expect from a wife whose husband revealed an illicit affair.

As Lyle saw it, he was trapped in a marriage to a woman who said she loved him but didn't care about his needs. She made him feel like a pervert for asking. He felt frustrated, rejected and whipped. In anger, he slowly built a case for why he was entitled to have oral sex with a stranger.

Now they were fighting over whether or not oral sex was sex. Since she always claimed it wasn't, Lyle said, he hadn't really cheated; if it was, then she'd been lying to him for all those years. He was smug and adamant; she couldn't change the rules on him now.

"What am I supposed to do?" Liz cried. "Are you going to divorce me because I don't like to give blowjobs? I should divorce you for cheating on me!"

I wasn't sure if they were fighting about his betrayal, about her inhibitions, or about whose definition was right. What I did know was that they loved each other and, despite their anger, wanted to save their marriage. I suggested they start small and see if they could renegotiate their erotic boundaries. They could start by talking about kissing: were some types of kisses better than others, how did they define a great kiss, what was their first kiss like, what was their best-ever kiss? Was it ever okay to kiss someone outside the marriage, or was all kissing reserved for each other? The exercise opened the door for them to begin exploring each other's sexual personality and needs more deeply.

Everyone defines sex slightly differently. Even if you were raised in the same place, went to the same school, and shared the same faith, don't make assumptions: develop a common sexual language with your partner. A recent study on levels of sexual well-being and satisfaction in marriages showed that couples who share the same attitudes about sex have the highest level of overall satisfaction in their relationships.

⊰ Chapter Six ⊱

The Best Reasons to Have Sex

———◄○►———

Humans have sex for a wide range of reasons, good and bad. However, study after study has shown that whenever people have sex for emotionally negative reasons, they also risk emotional trauma and physical illness. Physical resistance to sex often results in harm, from external bruising to internal tissue damage. Emotional resistance usually results in psychological pain. As previously elaborated, **consent matters**.

From a whole-body/mind health perspective — what works best for humans on a biological level, and what seems to maintain their best emotional balance — is eagerness for sex. A lot of the sexual science suggests that the more sincerely people want an encounter, the better the sex feels, emotionally, spiritually, and physically.

Below, are my models for the healthiest reasons why people have sex.

Sex for Pleasure

Pleasure and relief are what all creatures — human and animal — seek from sex. Sex, quite simply, is a human experience unlike all others. Good sex is good for us. In the bliss of passion, we feel more alive, more powerful. Sex gives us exciting glimpses at our primal selves. Sex inspires spiritual feelings and a unique emotional bond with our partner. When we're in love, the bonding may make us feel as if we've merged into one sacred entity with our partner. But even when sex is solo or casual, it still brings waves of intensely pleasurable feelings. To my mind, having sex because it makes you feel wonderful is the most positive expression of human sexuality possible.

Sexual tension weighs on us heavily, distorting our moods, impairing self-esteem, diminishing optimism. Despite the propaganda that sublimation is an effective way to relieve sexual tension, only the physical release of sex and orgasm can relieve sexual tension. That's right! Amazing but true, you cannot relieve sexual tension by any other method except by relieving sexual tension! It isn't brain science, though we have the brain science to prove it. Sublimation works to defer the impulse but the body still craves its thrilling brain chemical cocktail of natural pain relievers and mood enhancers. The more people repress and thwart that natural sexual drive, the greater their risk of mental and physical illness.

Sex for Reproduction

Consciously trying to have a baby can be a profoundly emotional, bonding act among humans. Although we now tend to plan families, or are at least aware when a woman is fertile and likely to conceive, for much of human history it was generally believed that gods (or God) decided when conception would occur. Fertility prayers have existed throughout recorded history. Our ancestors had as much sex as possible in hopes that the heavens would smile favorably on a night's union.

Still, if we weren't wired for pleasure, reproduction would be a dreary and taxing proposition. The notion that reproduction is the primary, or superior, reason why people have sex is a moral position, not a scientific one. In the upcoming section on sexual intercourse, I'll afflict you with the reasons and history behind this morality. For now, suffice to say, reproductive sex has its own important virtues and benefits, but being "the best" or "the real" reason people have sex are not among them.

In emotional and psychological terms, the period of consciously trying to make a baby — in other words, deliberately engaging in intercourse in hopes of creating new life — is perhaps one of the most emotionally meaningful experiences of adult life. For most adults, it's a time of optimism, faith, passion, tenderness, and a deepening commitment. Perhaps most of all it unites couples in a sacred purpose to do and create something greater than themselves: a family.

Sex for Physical and Mental Health

You've already read my lists of the health benefits of masturbation and orgasm. The role of sexual health — a functional libido, toned and healthy sex organs, good circulation in the pelvic region, a positive attitude towards sex — in human health cannot be overemphasized. Studies have shown that sexual pleasure and satisfaction are a key to human longevity and overall health, both physically and mentally.

Very slowly, some governments are beginning to catch on. In 2010, the Health Minister of Brazil publicly recommended that his country-people have more sex to combat the nation's alarming problems with high-blood pressure. It is one of the most intelligent pieces of advice any government official has even given, second only to Dr. Jocelyn Elders' endorsement of masturbation as a natural practice that could prevent unsafe sex — a comment considered so controversial in 1994, that then-President Clinton fired her for speaking the truth.

In my practice, I've seen the miracles wrought by improved sex lives, including clients overcoming chronic depression and symptoms of fibromyalgia by revitalizing their sex lives. So even when individuals aren't "in the mood" or have conditions which interfere with their ability to perform, I still urge them to find ways to climax. Sexual health usually tracks physical health: when one declines, the other usually follows.

Sex for Love

A lot of people give lip-service to sex by calling it lovemaking but not nearly as many people treat it as a genuine act of love. That is an opportunity missed. Sex is not only a beautiful expression of love and affection but, for many people, the most meaningful one.

I've occasionally worked with spouses who say, "Why does it always have to be about sex with my partner?" Usually, the simple answer is that the partner derives the deepest affirmation of love through acts of sex — not through the words one says, the money one earns, or the laundry one does. For some, that blowjob or that finger in their anus is more emotionally and spiritually meaningful than all the Valentine's cards in the world. Whether or not it "should" be that way is immaterial; it is that way for many people, and is neither a function of their morality or spirituality, but of their biological makeup.

The emotional hunger for intimacy runs deeper than the conscious mind. Sexual love has healing powers. It may smooth over arguments, put the day's petty woes behind us, bring us to a place of relaxation and tenderness, boost our spirits, and satisfy our need to belong to something greater than ourselves, such as an intimate coupling.

We all know how lousy we feel when we feel sexually rejected or treated like an object in bed. We know that people who treat sex as a duty never derive complete satisfaction from it (and neither do their partners). Clinically, I've observed that adults who are chronically ambivalent about their partners, emotionally closed off from them, or otherwise emotionally blocked experience the least overall satisfaction with their erotic interactions.

Sex for love has the opposite affects. It is emotionally reparative, ego-boosting, nurturing, and life-affirming to feel eagerly and fully embraced by someone you love. It's also incredibly hot. Literally. Love warms us up and promotes blood flow that warms our bodies, head to toe.

Love inspires a whole-body eagerness to have sex. When we love our partner, we crave to be in their arms and can't feel fulfilled until we feel their bodies against ours. A beloved's kiss may inspire feelings no one else in the world can give us. A mind filled with love and readiness, and a body warm and open to sexual experience, is in the perfect state to experience sexual ecstasy.

❧ Chapter Seven ❧

Sexual Intelligence

────◆◇◆────

You're probably familiar with the concept of "emotional intelligence," which measures intelligence according to behavior: the more intelligent your life choices, and the better your ability to learn from mistakes, the more rational your responses to emotional situations, the higher your emotional intelligence quotient. In the same vein, I view Sexual Intelligence as the ability to make wise, rational choices about your sex life: choices which produce satisfying, emotionally rewarding outcomes. Sexual intelligence and sexual health go together: you can't have one without the other.

Sexual immaturity and irrational, irresponsible sexual behavior are plagues in this culture. Throughout American society, adults behave childishly about sex, unable to discuss the subject calmly, even with the person they're having it with. People marry because they confused lust with love. Or they naively believe that a marriage license comes with a guarantee of sexual compatibility, and that sex will somehow magically "work itself out" once you enter your honeymoon suite. Unwanted pregnancies, STDs, sexual frustration, date rape, and a thousand other social dysfunctions are pervasive in our culture. It does not have to be that way.

As I said at the start of this section, if you can't talk about sex, you can't think about it. Now I'll add to it that with if you can't talk about sex, or think about it lucidly, you will never develop the Sexual Intelligence necessary to reach your full adult sexual potential.

Below are my theories on sexual intelligence in adults, broken down into its chief characteristics.

Characteristics of Sexual Intelligence

1. Self-Control

Everyone may give into an impulse now and again but if you have a pattern of sleeping with people you didn't plan to sleep with, engaging in risky behaviors or unsafe sex, or letting sex damage the quality of your non-sex life (work, family, relationships, finances), you have not yet developed the maturity and skill to put sexuality into its proper perspective in life.

Self-control is not the opposite of creative or spontaneous sex. It is the opposite of unsafe sex. Sexually intelligent adults develop a framework which allows them to indulge in wild hot sex while still maintaining control over their choices of partners, circumstances, and personal safety.

2. The Ability to Learn From Mistakes

One of the oddest things about we humans is our ability to deny reality. (The second oddest is that we always think it's the other guy who's in denial, but I'll save that for another book.) Sexologically speaking, denial is the devil that messes up many a sex life. Denying, for example, that you're having a sex problem when you are, in fact, having a sex problem never leads to a pretty outcome.

It is only by learning from your sexual mistakes and doing different or better next time, that you will grow.

I had a tedious boyfriend in my torrid 20s. No matter how many times I tried to guide his hand or explain I preferred gentle touches during foreplay, he always ended up clawing at my labia like a drowning man reaching for a life preserver. Beyond the Ouch Factor, it maddened me that he seemed to forget, from one night to the next, all my helpful suggestions on what would turn me on. As a therapist, I've discovered that this phenomenon is a lot more common than I suspected. In my office, it takes hundreds of forms. I've had any number of male clients who continuously visited sex-workers even though they felt horrible afterwards almost every time. Some of them felt bad before, during and after their visit, yet they still went to a sex-worker when they felt horny. I've had quite a few female clients who believed they were only entitled to orgasms if a man gave it to them: they would go for weeks, months and even years without orgasms, even though it made them miserable. And, of course, there are men and women who, for one reason or another, will feign ignorance of what their partner likes and wants in bed.

I'm thinking specifically of a male client whose wife pretended she didn't understand what he meant when he asked for a blowjob. She would give it a quick close-mouthed kiss and ask if that was enough. It would take him an hour to coax her into taking it into her mouth — a process he would have to repeat the next time he wanted fellatio. But there was also the woman whose husband initiated sex in the same exact and, to her, deeply irritating way. No matter how many times she asked him not to suddenly grasp her breasts tightly to signal that he wanted to sleep with her, he would keep grasping. In both cases, my clients were reduced to nervous wrecks by their partners' apparent stubborn resistance to ever giving them any sensual joy.

Sometimes the resistance is symptomatic of an underlying behavioral disorder. In my practice, I've observed that people previously diagnosed with Obsessive Compulsive Disorder and Attention Deficit Disorder, in particular, express those issues in their sexual behaviors. The adults I've treated who had been diagnosed as having ADD, for example, might be able to learn how to avoid a specific situation, but when a similar situation arose, they couldn't carry the lesson over because there were small changes in details or circumstance that made it feel like a new experience to them.

A person with Narcissistic Personality Disorder may subconsciously resist doing anything that they feel someone is demanding of them. They are primarily intersted in how *they* feel, not how their partner feels.

More often, a learning block in bed stems from an emotional issue, such as anger, which makes the person secretly resentful about making an effort to sexually please a partner. Others feel too emotionally fragile to change their behaviors — they may be sexually inhibited or shy, have a history of trauma or a deep sense of insecurity.

Unfortunately it isn't enough to know what one should or could do better; it's only by doing better that you are going to see better results. Flexibility and adaptability, and a mature commitment to learning as you go, are essential tools in every sexually intelligent lover's toolbox. In my perfect sex world, by the age of 40, all adults would be magnificently skilled lovers, adept at pleasing and being pleased by their partner of choice.

3. A Balance Between Body and Mind

Sexual intelligence requires a balance between what you know and what you feel. In other words, what you think about someone and what you feel for them erotically should function harmoniously, whether it's a one-night stand or a permanent, committed relationship. Studies have repeatedly proven that feeling united in body and mind not only results in the best sex but is mentally healthiest for you.

Of course, no one's perfect. We all have confusing relationships or experiences, or may blow hot and cold about someone. It's chronic in hormonal teenagers, and adults are equally prone to irrational sexual behaviors. But, barring any pivotal life crises (divorce, death of a loved one, depression over aging — *AKA* mid-life crisis — major illness or injury) which can send any of us into a tailspin of bad decision making, most adults reach a place of peace in their sexuality by middle age.

When your mind and body are at war over sex, the conflict manifests in numerous ways. It may diminish libido or impact performance; or, conversely, it can cause people to behave neurotically, expressing violent emotions or prompting them to engage in mindless or risky promiscuity. The greater the conflict, the more negative its outward expression is likely to be.

A recent study published in the *Archives of Sexual Behavior* suggests that this mind/body split is "the norm for women." I have theories about that which I'll address more specifically in the section on female sexual health, but suffice it to say that, indeed, women are more likely than men to have barriers between what they think about sex and what they feel about sex in bed because, on the whole, women tend to be more sexually inhibited than men.

Perhaps the most benign form of a mind/body split is when people's thoughts stray during sex — they may start thinking about housework or the bills during sex. Most often the culprits there are fatigue, boredom or stress. If it's circumstantial or occasional, it's not a problem. Chronic and severe dissociation, however, is indicative of much deeper psychological conflicts. In some cases, I've had clients who said their genitals feel almost numb when touched or that sexual stimulation feels unpleasant, "too intense," and otherwise puts them on edge. A few have described out-of-body-like experiences and the eerie feelings of watching themselves have sex.

Chronic sexual dissociation, in my opinion, requires insight/talk therapy to determine the underlying causes. As a rule of thumb, the greater the degree of dissociation in bed, the more likely it may have a pharmacological component (such as anti-depressants), which means a trip to a psychiatrist may be on the agenda. In my clinical experience, the causes for chronic dissociation have been post-traumatic stress, usually to a prior sexual trauma (rape or molestation), or a profound conflict about gender or sexual identity.

Happily, for most people struggling with intermittent blocks, or coping with inhibitions that impair their ability to get their minds and their bodies on the same page, numerous approaches have proven successful:

Meditation or faith-based practice which emphasizes a spiritual approach to holistic sexuality. I never specify the path people should take, as I feel each person's sexual choices should reflect their individual path in life, whether it is Christian, pagan or something else. Finding a place of peace is integral to developing balance.

Bodywork which explores and expands your ability to touch and be touched is an excellent method for reconnecting your mind to your sensuality. There are workshops and seminars throughout North America which offer couples and singles intensive work on expanding their sensual boundaries in a secular context, from "cuddle parties" to masturbation workshops. If you don't have access to such courses, try yoga. While it won't directly address your sexuality, yoga improves body confidence, builds better body image, and greatly enhances harmony between body and mind.

Therapy, counseling, peer therapy, group therapy, or Internet support groups all offer the information, insights, and support to help you deal with your particular obstacle. The deeper the problem, the more professional the help you should seek out. If you are having trouble focusing in bed because of stress, a therapist or life coach can get you through the problem. If you were abused, molested, or raped, insight therapy will help you heal. If your problems are complicated by addictions, poor impulse control, or conditions like OCD, ADD, Turret's, or bipolar disorder, make sure you keep up with your medications and get counseling to build coping skills. If you're bored with the sex you're having, see above about reaching new definitions and boundaries with your partner and read below for the section on honesty and its importance in a healthy, intelligent sex life.

4. Deliberate Choice

One of the most common issues I deal with in my practice is that a rather amazing number of people have sex for reasons other than pleasure. They have sex to compensate for inadequacies, to escape tedium, to win a bet, to prove a point, because they have nothing better to do, because their partner wanted it, because they feel guilty if they don't. Personal pleasure often is a distant priority in the convoluted passages of their souls.

The deliberate choice to have sex means that you are having sex because you expect it will make you feel good. It sounds simple. It should be. But it isn't.

As I explained earlier, the biological drive to have sex for pleasure is within us all. Pleasurable sex is human nature's own wonder drug: it eases the pain of life with its super-blend of brain chemicals. It reduces aggression, combats depression, and is a preventative to many diseases. When people have sex for reasons other than pleasure, they don't seem to reap the full benefits of that happy blend. Instead, they seem to lose touch with human sexual programming which naturally seeks a positive, relaxing form of release.

I've worked with many individuals who were angry that their partners never gave them what they needed in bed. They described their partners as "selfish" and "withholding," and they likely were; but it was also apparent that my clients shared responsibility for the relationship dysfunction. They didn't speak up about their own needs and expectations. They let their partners dictate all the rules. They waited for their partners either to initiate or to give them the go-ahead. More often than not, their passivity stemmed from the secret belief that they were not entitled to the joys and pleasures that other people got from sex. From personal and clinical experience, I know that people who expect sex to feel good, and who felt entitled to get what they need from their one-and-only, usually have full, happy sex lives with their partners of choice.

In my practice, I put a lot of effort into helping clients "power up" and take charge of their own sexual destinies so that they can break out of the passivity of resigning themselves to a dis-satisfying sex life. If you expect sex to be difficult, ultimately it will become a self-fulling prophecy.

5. Self-Respect

If you've ever wondered why some people get partners who give them everything they want in bed and others end up with withholding, unaffectionate, or judgmental ones, the difference may be attributed to one's sexual self-image. If you don't believe that sex "matters" or that your body is sacred, chances are you will accept and even resign yourself to sexual dissatisfaction. (At the dark end of the spectrum, some people perpetually gravitate to partners who sexually mistreat or abuse them.) It's a vicious cycle: resigning yourself to an unhappy sex life erodes your self-respect and causes you either to stay with a partner who mistreats you or to pick the same selfish partner again and again. In the process, your ability to make intelligent choices is crushed.

Sexual self-respect implies that you select partners who respect you, and who believe that your sexual satisfaction is as important as their own.

With self-respect should come respect for your partner and his or her needs. In the best of all possible worlds, two sexually intel-ligent people treat each other as precious entities who can fulfill our deepest needs, and treasure that capacity by demonstrating compassion and attentiveness in bed. In fact, for most adults, the respect for your partner is a measure of your own self-respect. If you look down on your partner, or think his/her needs are "sil-ly" or "dirty," and you're sleeping with them, what does that say about you?

6. Anticipation of Pleasure

The expectation of pleasure is often the difference between people with great sex lives and people with mediocre or lousy ones. Those who look forward to sex as a positive, life-affirming experience are more receptive to overtures and more likely to initiate.

Another of my infinite clinical mantras is that "**anxiety is the antithesis of sexy.**" If, under the surface, you are afraid of intimacy, embarrassed about your body, inhibited about the odors and noises of sex, worried that you won't live up to someone's expectations or that they won't live up to yours, your natural ability to anticipate the pleasure of sex will be impaired. Instead of feeling happy on the inside about romantic connections, you may feel threatened by them or even resentful because they stir up your own conflicts. I've had dozens of clients who complained because their partners push their hands away and do not reciprocate a passionate kiss. It was not the sex per se the partners rejected, it was the roller-coaster of conflicted emotions that went along with the sex.

Repeatedly engaging in sex that doesn't really turn you on, which you didn't fully consent to, or which makes you feel worse about yourself almost invariably re-enforces fears and inhibitions about sex that make the next encounter even more psychologically complicated. Over time, people who don't expect pleasure from sex become more fragile, more fractured, may find themselves sexually dissociating (unable to concentrate on the sex they are having), or swearing off sex altogether to escape the inner turmoil. Sexual intelligence requires that you find a place of peace with sex and see it as a positive experience in life.

7. Predictable Positive Outcomes

Sex is great when it's spontaneous, when passion ignites, when the chemistry is perfect and you go a little wild. That said, every adult should have good boundaries and, more importantly, stick to them. Too much spontaneity in sex usually leads to regrets, diseases, and unwanted pregnancies. The hallmark of intelligent sex is some measure of predictability: knowing what parts of you respond best to what kind of stimulation; having a reasonable certainty that if you do those things you will have a wonderful time; and not ending up doing things that make you kick yourself the next day.

Here is my list of three essential aspects of predictably positive good experiences:

1. Emotionally bonded sex

I've worked with people who boast of the notches on their belt, but who nonetheless fail to maintain stable, rewarding relationships with any of their conquests. Yes, they had sex with a lot of people — but how good was it? The amount of experience you have is meaningless if all of that experience is third rate. In every case, the more we unraveled their romantic history, the grimmer the picture grew of transient relationships, one-night stands, poor communication and petty fights.

Although the data remain inconclusive for now, numerous studies have shown that human behavior is driven as much by our innate social instincts and emotional needs as by our biological or physical ones. Our personalities naturally encompass a network of interconnected social dependencies: a need for personal affirmation (feeling understood and accepted), a need to belong to a group or family, a need for tenderness (often expressed as grooming in our primate relatives), a need for sexual release with a partner, and so on.

In my clinical experience, it is blatantly obvious that people who feel some passion and affection for their lovers are mentally healthier and make much smarter sexual choices than those who have little or no feelings beyond an urge to merge with strangers. The emotional and spiritual components of sex are at least as important to human satisfaction as the physical act. I have observed that people who mainly have a history of unemotional sex remain emotionally stunted and immature in their sexuality and in their ability to build committed, responsible relationships. Repeatedly placing your body into strange, uncomfortable, unpredictable sexual situations will take a toll on both self-esteem and emotional stability.

That said, the depth of the bonding is as fluid as the people and their relationship. There does not appear to be any one type of bonding that is better than another, as long as the experience is emotionally fulfilling. I was always fond of Eric Clapton's musical exhortation to "love the one you're with." It is an excellent bit of Zen wisdom: be where you are when you are there.

2. Honesty

As a therapist, I consider it part of my job to put myself out of a job. Sometimes, when I explain to clients that my hope is that one day they can tell their partner some of the sexual secrets they tell me, they'll exclaim, "You can't expect me to tell him/her THAT! What will he/she think of me?"

Usually, by the time our work is done, they are ready to tell their partners — and, more than that, to expect that their needs and desires will be taken seriously. How do you go from being embarrassed to whisper stuff to your sex therapist to announcing to your partner that you want to be screwed every day or cross-dress on Sundays? I think it comes, really, from believing that your truth matters, in bed as much as anywhere else, and that the person who loves you will learn to fit your needs into the greater context of a positive, fulfilling relationship.

It baffles me that so many adults never tell the people they plan to spend their whole lives with what they really want in bed. Stranger still, this is a norm most Americans defend, as if keeping your sexual fantasies and desires secret from the person you are closest to is a good thing. But who are you really protecting? Is it our partner's delicate sensibilities which must be shielded from knowing we'd like to try an anal probe or is it our own shame over wanting the things we want? I don't think we need to communicate every single sex fantasy we have or constantly report on our sexual thoughts. But if you can't tell your nearest and dearest what you want in bed, you may end up cheating yourself and them out of sexual happiness.

As a therapist, I have seen all the permutations. Some people are married to prudes who engage in high drama of the fainting-couch variety when they discover their partner's perversions. Usually because of religious or political beliefs, some adults think it's better to be divorced than to remain married to someone whose sexuality they consider immoral. But most adults are willing, at least, to listen and make some compromises when it's someone they sincerely care about.

More often, it is the person with the fantasy who censors him or herself for fear of being rejected or mocked. Almost everyone who came to me claiming their partner would never accept them "if they only knew" what their secret fantasies were discovered that, in fact, their partners were much less perturbed by their inclinations than they were. I've never met a spouse who felt good about their partner lying to them or cheating on them, but the weird fantasies themselves are generally much less of a problem. This has, in my experience, been especially true of fetishists: after spending a lifetime of feeling stressed or ashamed of what many fetishists perceive as a fundamental defect in their personality, they may become invested in protecting someone they love from seeing them as they see themselves, i.e., ugly and flawed.

Perhaps the most bittersweet example was an elderly man who contacted me on the brink of despair. He had fantasized about spankings his entire life, but never once in 45 years of marriage, had he confessed them to his wife. He thought that part of his fantasy life had long-since died — until the Internet came along with its myriad temptations to re-light the spanking fire in his aging loins. He was both horrified at the possible results of telling her, but gripped by a need so real and now, after decades of repression, so great he feared he would end up cheating on her if he did not.

Because they were at a crisis point in their marriage, we worked intensively over several consecutive days. In the course of that time, he told his wife everything; his wife acted shocked, angry and hurt, and emotionally shut down on him; he plunged into worse despair; she mentioned the D-word (divorce); he grew angry, and echoed the D-word back at her; and finally, she shyly admitted she'd fantasized about dominating him and forcing him to service her orally, and asked if he would give her more oral sex if she spanked him. He quickly assured her he would be delighted to do so, especially after a spanking. I could see in their eyes that both of their minds were now racing with a whole new world of erotic fantasies. In the course of one very emotionally grueling week, they changed the course of their intimacy, and reached a level of passion neither had imagined possible at their age.

I can only imagine what their lives together might have been like if they'd both been honest about their sexual fantasies from the beginning, but I firmly believe it's never too late for the truth to set you free.

3. Sobriety

In a culture which celebrates the use of alcohol and drugs, sex and intoxication seem to go hand in hand. The extra buzz of a mild intoxicant can enhance sensual and even sensation. I've occasionally advised couples to sip a glass of red wine or other "soft" stimulant together to help them warm up and relax sexually. However, there's a big difference between moderate use of mild stimulants to arouse your senses and getting bombed, which generally numbs everything, including your intelligence.

Once you blur your ability to make good decisions, all bets are off as to whether you will get through your sexual experience safe and sound. If your judgment is significantly compromised, you may agree to things you'd never do if you were in your right mind; you may forget or neglect (or just become too stupid) to use protection against STDs. In sufficient doses, alcohol and drugs may make you feel so good you don't know when something is hurting or endangering your health, a leading reason why some people end up in emergency rooms after sex.

Of all the drugs popular in North America, alcohol is the most ubiquitous legal drug, and therefore the most dangerously abused. Alcohol is the common culprit behind impotence, bad sex, sexual injuries/accidents, aggressive sex, rape, and sexual battery. In my clinical opinion, if you MUST be stoned out of your mind to enjoy sex, you shouldn't have sex again until you find a path to sobriety, whether it's through counseling or a hard look at yourself in the mirror of reality.

⊰ꗃ Chapter Eight ꗃ⊱

Sex Problems Are Life Problems

————⟨○⟩————

I have all kinds of sexological mantras I inflict on clients, basic rules of thumb that I want them to remember, such as **"anxiety is the antithesis of sexy"** and **"an orgasm a day keeps the doctor away."** Another is **"what happens in the bedroom isn't just about the bedroom."** What I mean by that, simply, is you can't completely separate the emotions in the bedroom from the way you act and feel about life in general. The reverse is true as well: if your interactions with your partner during the day are rocky, your sex life may suffer.

Every fight, every resentment or grudge, every insecurity or fear which causes you personal stress may come back to haunt you when you get into bed. Depending on your or your partner's own patterns of expressing stress, this can go either way: some people have more sex when they're fighting because it's a way to escape from their real-world problems; some people shut the sex valve off and retreat from intimacy when they're upset. One of the reasons make-up sex feels so exciting is because it brings resolution — through sex — to the emotional conflict.

In my clinical experience, the people who seem to suffer the most from performance problems, for example, often feel neglected, criticized or judged by their partners. After a day of browbeating in the living room, the bedroom may feel like a minefield. It's hard to let yourself feel vulnerable and open to a partner you don't emotionally trust.

I've learned that, for many people, sex is not really about sex but about reams of other, often unresolved, issues in their lives. Female performance, for example, can hinge on issues like body image; women who are embarrassed about their genitalia, or dissatisfied with their breast size, for example, may express those anxieties in the bedroom. It can, as I commonly see in therapy, make them reluctant to engage in sex, uneasy about being naked, unable to allow themselves to be vulnerable during the act of sex. Sometimes poor body image can lead to people acting out in sexually self-destructive ways — mindless promiscuity, risky or unsafe sex, or — at the other extreme — asexuality and fear of sex.

The ebb and flow of sexual emotions are with us at all times, even when we aren't conscious of them. As I've said before, the repression of sexual feelings alone exacts a price in terms of stress. The more stress we feel, the less sensual we feel, and the more separated we feel from others. People who feel unloved or under-valued may demonize a partner's sexual fantasies or needs, throwing up roadblocks to honest communication about what's really bothering them. People who use sex as a weapon to hurt or humiliate their partners inflict the most emotional damage of all. People who grow sexually alienated from their partners tend to withdraw into themselves. In my observation, some couples who fight bitterly over money or issues of fairness in the relationship are really angry because one of them feels unfairly treated in bed. If, night after night, something is off in bed, your growing mistrust and resentment will jade your faith in your partner and compromise your sexual performance as well.

I've seen both ends of the spectrum: couples who fight bitterly over a sex act or an unusual request from their partner, blaming everything that is wrong in their relationship on the sex. I've seen couples, like Leon and Patrice B, who fought over everything except their most significant problem: an inability to communicate in bed.

Leon and Patrice came to me during a bad patch in their relationship, worried that if it got much worse, they'd end up divorced. Patrice was tired of Leon's gruff, seemingly indifferent behavior.

Leon saw Patrice as a shrew, who constantly criticized him and reminded him of every mistake he'd ever made. During their first session, they interrupted and corrected each other so many times, they worked themselves into a screaming fight. Then Leon grew silent and moody and withdrew, which sent Patrice into a rage. They bickered over everything — how they met, who did more of the chores, who was more loyal. Every minute aspect of their relationship was subject to quarrelsome debate. The only thing they seemed to agree about was that both of them were unhappy.

When I asked about their sex life, they said that they currently did not have one. They had both lost all interest in each other. After what I'd just witnessed, I was not surprised. I asked if they had had good sex in the past. Both grudgingly admitted they had, that it was one of the best parts of their marriage. But about a year ago, things changed, and Leon now spent more nights on the living room sofa than in their bed. They both assured me it was better that way, at least for now.

When I asked if either of them knew what had caused the change in their sex life a year earlier, Patrice said she had no idea and Leon grew quiet. It took a private session with him to finally get him to admit that ever since their last child was born, Jean had wanted less and less sex. It had gotten to the point where he was lucky to get a hand-job a couple of times a week. He was able to live with that, he said, but then one night Patrice announced that she had enough pressure in her life, and wished he'd stop pushing her for sex. They'd been married for 13 years at that point. He was so hurt by this rejection, he decided that she probably had never liked having sex with him, and that she had silently resented him the whole time.

He said that for the first week thereafter, he was so upset he didn't think he would be able to perform, even if she wanted it. She acted relieved that he had backed off, so he let it go. So did she. After a few weeks he realized it was easier simply to push sex away from his mind and focus on their child, who was now the best part of the marriage, as far as he was concerned. He treated his wife as a roommate, he stopped asking for sex, and they stopped being intimate. After a few months, she finally approached him, saying they hadn't been together for a while, and she was in the mood.

Instead of feeling grateful, as he would have in the past, he was angry that it had taken her so long to notice they weren't having sex. He shrugged off her overture, believing she was only offering because she was afraid he might leave her.

When I spoke privately with Patrice, she told me her version. Leon was always pushing her for sex. He wanted to have it three times a day. She didn't mind when they first married but since having children, she didn't have the energy or interest to do it that often. Meanwhile, she loved when Leon held her and kissed her but he didn't seem to want to do it unless he could then have sex with her. That only made her feel worse, as if she had to put out for him just to earn some scrap of affection.

Where once they had the outlet of sex to take the edge off their marital tensions — and the comforts of intimacy, the expression of love, the renewal and acknowledgment of passion between them — now they only had their anger, resentment, and mistrust. Leon never told Patrice how hurt he felt by her confession. Patrice never told him that she needed more cuddle-time. She also admitted she flipped off about the hand-jobs after a tense evening. She regretted her words the minute they left her mouth, but she feared that if she retracted them, he'd go back to pushing her for sex. So she too had come to accept their sexless marriage.

From my perspective, their inability to communicate their needs and be honest in bed had created an emotional divide in their lives outside of bed. They both walked around under a shadow of guilt, resentment, and hurt. This, in my opinion, led to all the pointless bickering and negative behavioral loop that threatened to destroy their emotional bond.

As I often point out to parents, one day your kids will grow up and leave home. If you spend the 20+ years it takes to raise children fighting with one another, what will you have when the children are gone? A really bad, sexless marriage, now unveiled as the mess it truly is.

I suggested that if they were serious about saving their marriage, they had to re-open the door to sexual intimacy. It is never too late to re-learn how to be exciting lovers. You may not be able to "recapture the spark" of early romance as so many sex columnists put it, but you can become romantic, caring adult sex partners, and people who know a lot more about giving and receiving pleasure than when you first paired up.

Sex can perform wonders for a couple: it can bond you; it can give you a period of time when you feel in complete harmony with someone else; it gives you the freedom to be vulnerable and safe; it brings physical comfort and relief, thanks to our amazing sexual biology; and most importantly it floods your mind and body with positive, loving energy and, after climax, a unique serenity.

In our three-way talks, I guided them to speak openly, for the first time, about all of their sexual expectations, disappointments, and desires. We began at the beginning, when they were first married: what were their hopes and dreams then, what were their sexual expectations and how had they evolved over time? As we slowly unraveled the history of their sex life together, they began to identify stress factors that had triggered sexual problems which, in turn, had led to arguments: when their kids were born; when Patrice's mother died; when Leon was studying for a licensing exam. During each of those periods, they would drift into fights and withdraw physically from each other. They hadn't perceived the pattern before, but once they did they began to realize that the problem was not the sex itself but their inability to manage stress in the marriage.

They also had to face the fact that they had different levels of libido. Leon was essentially unchanged from his youth, and Patrice's drive had diminished as a result of pregnancy and aging. There is no cure for a couple whose libidos are so different, only a choice to make a healthy compromise that both parties can live with. Maybe if Patrice got more affection and tenderness, she would be more willing to indulge him; meanwhile, if Leon's needs could be treated as valid and real, perhaps she could find less tiring but mutually enjoyable ways to be intimate with him.

As they rebuilt their marriage, Leon and Patrice started connecting the dots. They took my advice and agreed to cuddle and kiss every night before going to sleep, whether or not they had sex. They also made a date each week to talk. The rule was that they had to talk about themselves; not the children, their jobs, or their relatives. I suggested they try to have orgasms together as often as possible, even if they didn't have the time or energy for full-on lovemaking. I'm a firm believer that if you can make the time to brush your teeth at night, you can make the time for a quickie.

Through intimacy in bed and a genuine dialogue of emotions and sensuality, they turned their marriage around, even though nothing in their outside circumstances changed. They learned to treat what happened in their bedroom with genuine respect, as something as important to a stable marriage as eating dinner together as a family or visiting with relatives. They didn't shrug off each other's dissatisfaction or their mutual responsibility in making their sex lives as pleasurable as possible. In a few months, they were doing better than they had imagined possible.

❧ Chapter Nine ❧

Biology is Destiny,
But Not the Way You May Think

---◦---

Nature v. Nurture

Nature versus nurture is the debate at the center of most public dialogue about sexual differences: are people born to be
(fill in the blank: gay, fetishistic, bisexual, transgendered) or is it
their raising (parenting, environment, culture) which shapes their
sexual identity? The answer is that it's both. Not a terribly satisfying answer to people who want black and white answers about
sex. Nonetheless, for now it's the only one we have and I suspect
it's the only one we ever will.

Our individual sexual identities are as complicated as our personalities, something else which cannot be absolutely predicted by
science. And, just like our personalities, our sexual identities are
the product of a complex and infinite range of variables that begin
with genetics and are continually shaped, modified, and transformed by life experiences and health circumstances from infancy
to old age.

Still, people keep hoping and longing for answers, and every generation has produced movements and theorists who believe they have unearthed a unified theory to define what normal, natural sex is or should be for every human being. In recent generations, Biological Determinists and Evolutionary Psychologists have pushed for a definitive context to frame gender and sexuality. Some of the scientific work has been excellent. We have proven again and again that biology plays a much larger role in human sexuality than previously expected. Modern science has more or less confirmed Krafft-Ebing's late 19th century speculation that humans are born, or "constitutionally disposed," towards particular sexual behaviors. He based his ideas on anecdotal and clinical experience. Now we have ample scientific data which demonstrate that sex drive and sexual responses are inherited traits, and that many human sexual behaviors (particularly mating behaviors) are universal, even when their cultural expressions take different forms.

Studies have shown that even when people have no idea they are being driven by a sexual impulse, their brains "think" differently. For example, while we don't think we're doing something sexual when we get prepared for a date, underlying biological forces are subconsciously informing our decisions on what to wear and how to groom. Every culture has beautifying rituals intended to improve a person's chances of finding a mate. It is difficult, of course, to separate a culture which promotes fashion and cosmetics from our innate biological urge to increase our chances for sex. Still, human psychology seems to instinctively know that the prettiest person gets the most sexual attention. The more options for sex, the more benefits, including the ability to choose the best partners for reproduction and to increase longevity through abundant and healthful sex.

However, that's where biological determinism must take a backseat to societal trends, personal morality, individual circumstances, and public health. If destiny was dictated by biology, then the most beautiful people should have the most desirable partners, have the most sex, and live the longest. In reality, beautiful people are not more or less likely than anyone else to achieve any of the preceding. Everything depends on how and where they were raised, what they were taught, their moral values, their religious beliefs, their self-esteem, their personal character, their expectations, their health status, their economic class, and — of course — luck and chance.

Meanwhile, thanks to modern medical technology, it's now possible for men and women to remain youthfully responsive into old age, even though our brain is wired to our reproductive clock. Biologically, most of us would be through with sex in our 50s and 60s. Happily, with hormone replacement therapies and ED drugs, and gigantic progress in public health, gerontology, endocrinology, and medicine in general, contemporary sexual behavior in people between the ages of 55 and 90 are breaking all the records in human history.

The large population of Baby Boomers is a driving force. Even the most conservative elements of our society were not immune from the transformative social philosophies of the free love 60s, the swinging 70s, and the profound impacts of the women's lib and gay rights movement on the American consciousness. Many who were prudes in their youth have now embraced their sexuality. Those delightfully 21st century concepts, MILFs, GILFs, and Cougars, reflect a monumental shift in underlying cultural perceptions of female sexuality and beauty. According to numerous studies, casual sex has become so common in retirement communities that the CDC views seniors as a higher-risk group for STDs than people in their 20s.

Perhaps my biggest beef with biological determinism though is that, at its heart, it imposes cultural assumptions on biological data. You may have read, for example, that women prefer men with lots of money because they need providers for their children; that women are all "mama lions" protecting their children, or that in the cave days men were brave, powerful hunters and women stayed close to the cave, gardening, cooking and taking care of babies. We all have an image of these primitive peoples forming pairs and monogamous relationships because, after all, every woman needed a man to provide for her, right?

I'm not saying these theories are impossible, only that they are highly implausible. In fact, at least one theory was recently proven false. A 2010 study with the dry title, "Sex Differences in Mushroom Gathering: Men Expend More Energy to Obtain Equivalent

Benefits," (Pacheco-Cobos, L. et al.), yielded data that suggests that men took to hunting because they were poor at cultivating crops and were, in a sense, pushed out of the "cave" by the ladies, who were far more accomplished at the essential skills that kept families consistently fed. Indeed, even in the most oppressive societies, women have always found ways to be financially independent.

It is literally impossible, even for this author, to remove the patriarchal assumptions from a patriarchy that has shaped values and beliefs for thousands of years. To assume that biological imperatives make all men one way and all women another way, without sexual or gender variations is to forget that there is life outside the laboratory of one's own mind. Some of the theories about "natural" sex roles among primitive humans are based on highly evolved social and religious dogma, not on archaeological records or other evidence that, in fact, people ever lived such black-and-white, "Ozzie and Harriet in loincloths" lives.

To understand biology versus destiny, we must look at the subject from an interdisciplinary and historical perspective. Diversity has always been the norm. There have always been transsexuals, homosexuals, lesbians, bisexuals, sex workers, cross-dressers, swingers, multiple marriages, polygamists, adulterers, fetishists, and sadomasochists throughout world cultures, in all times and places. Prostitution has long been called "the oldest profession in the world" for good reason: transactional sex (giving some form of payment or reward in exchange for sex) has been observed among primates, and recent studies suggest it is hardwired into humans. Archaeological evidence suggests that Stone Age forebears exchanged trinkets for sexual favors, and has amply demonstrated that the same sexual behaviors we see today are as old as recorded history, which in turn suggests they existed prehistorically as well.

For an edited glimpse of human sexual behavior among the ancients, we don't have to look any further than the Old Testament, where polygamy, polyamory, prostitution, pedophilia, sexual slavery, and a host of perversions (Lot's incest with his daughter, King Solomon's fetishistic sex with his concubines, and Abraham's adultery with a slave girl, to name but a few) are condoned by the

Almighty. Mary Magdalene figures large in the New Testament, a prostitute who was treated with compassion and understanding by Jesus Christ.

Nor were gender roles ever cut and dried, though civilizations attempted to organize them by sex, assigning biological males to one group of endeavors and biological females to another. In most Euro-centric societies, transpeople were generally marginalized or compelled to conceal their identities. Still, now and again individuals or groups emerged who defied even the most rigid cultural standards. History books are filled with examples of women who publicly dressed and lived as men, including medieval saint, Joan of Arc and that icon of the American Wild West, Calamity Jane. Transsexed people have existed in all times and places, their social position dependent on period and culture. In South Asia, the cult of the Hijra (male-to-female trans person) has been known since the Moghul empire. Theirs is a long and tragic history marred by oppression and marginalization. However, in North America, the "Two-Spirit" (male and female) person was a figure of respect among an estimated 130 Native American tribes, and performed specific social duties, including healing, prophecy and religious functions.

And so it goes, all the way down the sexual line. Throughout history, some cultures allowed sexual non-conformists to thrive, while others clamped down on their social freedoms or restricted them to special professions or confined them to certain districts. In some Greco-Roman and Middle Eastern cultures, it was an accepted custom — even a badge of pride — for wealthy married men to keep young male lovers on the side. In the 21st century, some of the same cultures which once accommodated gay liaisons are now virulently homophobic.

A final factor influences sexual behaviors: the sheer force of history. Perhaps the most dramatic example in modern history happened in Berlin, Germany between 1920 and 1940. 1920s Berlin was a cultural mecca for sexual free-thinkers and non-conformists. Nudist (Naturist), libertine, gay, lesbian, bisexual and cross-dressing cultures flourished there. For a moment in time, a new, progressive attitude towards human sexuality emerged from the dark ages of Victorianism. That all changed when the Nazis came to power in the 1930s and embarked on a reign of terror against sexual nonconformists. With the burning of the vast research collection amassed by sexological pioneer Magnus Hirschfeld in 1933, the Nazis set about a decade-long crusade against any sexual material that did not promote Hitler's plan to create a so-called superior race by impregnating all available "pure Aryan" women. To Nazi eyes, anything which promoted sex for pleasure was decadent and "un-German." Soon, the same landlords and restaurant owners who once warmly greeted their lesbian and gay patrons became collaborators, who turned them in to the Gestapo. Untold numbers of homosexuals and bisexuals were shipped to concentration camps. In just 20 years, Germany went from being one of the most sexually enlightened societies in the world to one of the most violently, institutionally repressive ones ever known.

As history changes, so do the ebb and flow of sexual attitudes. Not only do we adapt to new situations, but our beliefs adapt as well. We can see it in the current dilemma over polygamy in the Mormon faith. "Plural marriage" (one man, several wives) has always been controversial within the Mormon Church. Despite harsh public criticism when Joseph Smith introduced plural marriage into Mormon faith in 1831, polygamy was openly embraced by several major Mormon leaders and became fairly common practice in Utah. Mainstream America remained opposed to Mormon plural marriage, and soon began enacting laws to limit the definition of marriage to one man and one woman. In 1862 the first national law against bigamy was passed, followed by numerous other laws and decisions that re-enforced monogamous marriage as the only legal form of marriage. In response to the legal atmosphere in the U.S., the Latter Day Saints (LDS) began issuing formal statements against plural marriage and, beginning in 1910, threatened excommunication, although it was known that many traditionalist Mormons continued their traditional plural marriages well into the mid 20th century. Today's mainstream Mormon shares the common American belief that a marriage is a monogamous union between man and woman. Polygamists who follow the traditions of the Mormon founders are now a marginalized and dispersed community (estimated at less than 20,000) who usually live under the radar to avoid arrest and prosecution.

Thus the doors of history open and close on sexual minorities and non-conformists. Depending on their society, they will either be visible or invisible; they will either be allowed to function openly or will go underground.

What would humans be like "in the raw" of our biological impulses and universal sexual desires? To obtain an unflinchingly real snapshot of human sexual biology, one must imagine humanity without religion, without civilization and social customs, without laws, without a developed language, and without education, money, or modern technology. In other words, sad to say, one must look at the bonobo. I'm sad because humans are so unlike other species that comparisons even to our closest biological relative are significantly flawed. That said, as our closest primate cousin, sharing 98% of our genetic material, the bonobo is our single best source for insights into what human sexuality might have been like in the wild, when homo sapiens first appeared on Earth. And, frankly, it's fucking frightening.

Bonobos are a notoriously omnisexual species: they use sex to enhance social affiliation (to express bonding, affection, friendship); to establish their status in the group; as a bartering and transactional tool; to sublimate violence and mitigate conflict; and, I suppose, mainly because it feels fantastic. For bonobos, almost any time is the right time for sex, with everyone, including their own young. Bonobos are rampantly promiscuous and bisexual. They masturbate alone, in couples, and in groups. Both sexes possess incredible sexual stamina and appetites. Male bonobos are relentless, amoral, perverted sexual opportunists. Female bonobos shriek for sex and become violent if their males-of-choice won't indulge their sexual appetites.

Sounds a little like that singles bar you once visited, right? But happily we are not bonobos who, indeed, are, as best we can tell, truly bound by their biological natures. We alone, as a species, do rise above out biological imperatives. So when it comes to biology versus destiny, I boil it down to one question: Given that variety is the norm, and understanding that without any social controls, we would be as unprepared for a normal functional human life as the average bonobo, where should we draw the lines between how we were made and how we should act?

Sexual Biology and Reality

As a sex therapist, my sole agenda is to help adults find a place of peace with their sexual identities and to guide them to make good choices, based on their individual beliefs, their personalities, their expressed needs, and their sexual identities. The goal is to find a balance in their sex lives that allows them to create a context for fulfilling their needs without causing harm either to themselves or others. When a Christian who believes in monogamy works with me, I don't suggest that he or she try swinging to spice things up. On the other hand, if I'm working with a polyamorous pagan, I'm not going to recommend they aim to be a good Christian. It is, in my opinion, all about building a meaningful, individualized context for your sexuality, and integrating your values outside of the bedroom with your sexual needs. As I often tell patients, a good sex therapist does not try to change you and make you act like someone else — a good one tries to help you to be the person you would be if you didn't have emotional issues like shame, self-doubt, or anxiety blocking your natural sexual responses.

My counseling philosophy makes me cynical to the point of anger at sex therapists (such as "aversion therapists" and religion-based counselors) who believe there is only one "normal" or moral type of sexual conduct between partners. I think we can all agree, more or less, on appropriate public sexual conduct, and there are laws governing that. But when it comes to what adults choose to do in private, there should be only one rule: it should make you feel good physically and emotionally.

Mutual consent sets sex free. If getting tied up and spanked is your idea of a perfect night with your partner, and your partner agrees, congratulations. If spending the evening enjoying a long session of oral sex with your honey is your vision of nirvana, and your partner agrees, have fun with it. If you need a fancy whap-doodle and want to dance around like a poodle, and your partner wants to be the ringmaster, so what? No one but your partner — whom, presumably, you trust with your secrets — will ever know. Sexual preferences carry no more intrinsic meaning than a person's choice in foods, clothes, music, or furniture.

I realize that my laissez-faire attitude towards private sexuality makes some people consider me a wild-eyed radical. I just see myself as extremely pragmatic. Sex is what it is. Diversity is the norm. People need and want different things. They always have. They always will. It's not my job to judge, even when I don't understand or am personally turned off by the scenarios they describe. It's my job to show them that being an adult means taking control over your sexual destiny. Adults can arrive at a solution, even if it is a compromised solution, that will achieve better, more satisfying results.

Social Limits and Sexual Harm

So when does a therapist have to say, "No, you can't do this?" For me, that boundary is like a wide white line painted down my brain: anything which causes unwanted pain or suffering to someone else. Sexual behavior which causes harm, sexual behavior which is not fully consented to by all involved, should be viewed as anti-social behaviors. For the good of all, anti-social sexual behaviors must be curbed, punished and, ideally, treated.

On my personal short list of anti-social sexual behaviors, I include pedophilia, deliberate infection with an STD, and any type of coercive, deceptive, or nonconsensual sexual behavior — from the extremes of rape and molestation to lesser offenses such as subway groping or secretly taping people nude or in sexual situations. Such behaviors reflect an inability to make moral choices or a lack of empathy for their victim that may be sociopathic. In other words, they intentionally cause harm or misery to others. Those who exhibit such anti-social behaviors are best treated by forensic sexologists and psychologists who specialize in criminal sexual behavior.

On the other hand, creating or enforcing laws to control the type of sex consenting adults enjoy, or prosecuting people who engage in unpopular sex (as opposed to criminal sex) is like banning anti-freeze because some people have used it to poison others to death. Sex is much safer than antifreeze. Sex is, in fact, beneficial. It is the sociopath who uses sex as a weapon who must be held responsible for his or her crime. Where no harm is done, no penalty is required.

On my short list of sexual behaviors that do not cause social harm but are, instead, simply a cause of discomfort or religious upset to a segment of American society, I include sex work (adult movies, prostitution, stripping, et al) and homosexuality. Despite innumerable studies and tracts which have attempted to convince the public that both are harmful to society, the only reliable data we have ever had shows the exact opposite: granting equal marriage rights to gays vastly improves local economies and legalized prostitution is not only a cash-cow to governments but also creates a positive sea-change in public health as well.

The US Government above all should understand the benefits of calmly regulating sex workers. In the wake of the bombing of Pearl Harbor, US military officials most efficiently ran the prostitute district of Hawaii, providing horny soldiers and sailors on leave with a safe environment for patronizing hookers.

Finally, some strong words about child molestation. In recent years, child molesters have been rationalizing their behaviors by saying, "We were born that way," and presenting themselves as an oppressed sexual minority, with comparisons to gays and lesbians. Personally, I do not believe child molesters are born: I believe they were traumatized in childhood and lost their capacity to empathize with the people they victimize. But even if data emerges at some point showing that a particular genetic anomaly leads to the formation of a pedophiliac personality, I would say that when you balance the risks and rewards of acting on that behavior, the only moral choice is indeed for the pedophile to learn how to suppress his or her sexual urges. When it comes to behaviors like rape or molestation, anti-social biology must either suppress its urges or face the social punishments meted out to those who commit harm.

The best case against allowing people with anti-social biology to run free is the biology of their victims. It is precisely because of our biology as children that sexual contact with adults can be so damaging (and, obviously, the more invasive the contact, the greater the damage). For one, as previously discussed, children don't have complete sexual feelings. Sex is NOT in their brains the way it is for an adolescent or adult; they have neither the right chemicals nor adequate knowledge and experience of their bodies to feel what adolescents and adults feel. Children, for example, do not fantasize about or desire sexual penetration. Children do not see or perceive sex the way grown-ups do. A recent study showed a vase decorated with an optical illusion called metamorphosis; if you're an adult, when you look at it, you see a couple in naked embrace; but when children look at the same design, they notice the little dolphins (which look like shadows to adults) swimming around, and the naked figures are an obscure background blur.

If biology must rule some piece of destiny, then the mental health of children absolutely trumps any adult's rights to have orgasms at their expense.

There really should be only one perfect biological model of natural sex: adults who want to give and receive pleasure with each other. That is the biology destiny I dream about.

⤜⊰ Afterword ⊱⤛

——⟨○⟩——

I recently read about the so-called "rampant promiscuity" of the female red squirrel. Apparently, the ladies copulate with as many as 14 different partners a day. Scientists looked for potential causes, and studied whether this behavior was inherited (it is not). Not finding some magic extra-horniness gene to explain the behavior, they remain bemused by the bushy-tailed strumpets who exceeded the reproductive imperative by mating with as many males as they could find.

Another article that intrigued me was the discovery that, when raised in a hot, humid climate, male butterflies are the aggressors in the game of love. However, when raised in a cool, dry climate, their roles reverse, and it is the female who pursues the male. One of the media reports pointed to this anomaly as proof that "species will do anything to reproduce."

Butterflies are not the only species which change gender roles (or even sex) in response to climate and environment. In some common species of fish, females will "change" their sex when there is a shortage of males. Studies of the fish in the Thames River in England have shown that water pollution is causing female mutations in male fish. In some species of birds, when females are unavailable, other males assume the wifely role. And, of course, in human beings, when opposite-sex partners are unavailable, same-sex relationships become a norm (witness our prison system, where homosexuality may become a survival mechanism).

I love quirky animal sex studies which offer glimpses into the breathtaking diversity of sex in its most natural state. Whatever squirrels and butterflies do, we can feel confident they do so from a natural impulse, and not because they saw it on the Internet or learned it at school. It reveals something profoundly honest about the universal nature of sex.

I find it frustrating, however, when the scientists performing the research or the journalists reporting it, demonstrate their un-natural bias. In this, it's often science reporters who are at fault for seeking out a spicy headline that twists the original studies' meanings or intentions. Perhaps the most infamous case was back in the 1990s when media reported that scientists had found a "gay gene," something the original scientists never claimed (nor found). Nonetheless, the news spread and many people believed the story, not simply because they saw it on the news, but because these people would like to have a definitive, concrete explanation for why people are gay.

Social expectations mar the overall reporting on sex. If, for ex-ample, we expect male animals always to be the hornier, more ag-gressive, or more dominant suitor, then aggressive or libidinous females will always be curiosities. If we assume that reproduction drives all sexual desire, then sex for fun will always seem anoma-lous. If we believe that gender is binary (all males are this, while all females are that), we will never get a realistic picture of the shades of gray between male and female. If we seek black and white answers, we will probably always be frustrated because sex is filled with anomalies and exceptions. Lines between gender, sexual orientation, and even libido can be blurry and permeable.

The idea that sexual behavior is driven by an overwhelming urge to reproduce is, simply put, religious by nature. Some may find it comforting to believe that the reason we have sex in the first place is because a divine force is pushing us to multiply towards some glorious divine goal, thus elevating sex beyond its biological function. That edict is debatable and best confined to theological speculation.

I think it's much more realistic and evidence-based simply to as-sume we are driven to have sex because we were born to be sexu-al, regardless of our desire or ability to reproduce. To believe that reproduction drives sex, and that sex therefore should purposeful and productive ignores the facts that most adult couples prefer non-reproductive sex.

Three sweeping categories of individuals are omitted from the reproductive norm in hurtful ways. The most obvious, of course, are the vast number of Americans who fit under the LGBT umbrella: lesbians, gay men, bisexuals, trangendered people, and queers. A smaller but meaningful minority are all the others of us who deliberately have sex for pleasure (whether it's fetish sex, kinky sex, swinging, group sex or tantric sex). While many of us who fall into those categories have kids, that's usually NOT why we have sex. Reproduction is the last thing on our minds when we think about a night of orgasmic fun.

The second group is all the people who, for one reason or another, cannot have biological children. I wonder if they feel as bad as gay people when their friends or clergy make it sound as if reproduction is the best or only reason to have sex. No wonder so many people who are physiologically unable to have children feel shame, self-doubt, and depression. If the value of a human life is pegged to its ability to reproduce, sterility renders your life worthless. That's how previous generations viewed it and tragically, it is often still regarded today.

The third group is women who are past their reproductive years. Thankfully, attitudes have shifted enormously throughout the 20th and 21st centuries but even in our mothers' and grandmothers' generations, women beyond the age of childbearing were generally considered asexual, undesirable and "finished" as women. One of the great secret tragedies of women's history, in my opinion, are the hundreds of millions of women who were discarded or disenfranchised once their childbearing years were done, and long before their need and desire for romance and intimacy had ebbed. While society remains uneasy about all the swinging grandmas and grandpas out there, the miraculous coincidence of a Baby Boomer generation and the Sexual Revolution of the 60s and 70s, has resulted in new generations of women who no longer believe that their sex and love lives must end at menopause.

Now, what if...? What if sex drive is not welded to reproduction in humans? What if sex exists primarily to help us remain cheerful, stress-free, and youthful? What if sex is a life-positive act, promoting better health, increasing longevity, and total wellness, a naturally programmed "self-cleaning" system of a sort that restores (rather than saps) vitality? What if reproduction is (for those who want kids) a blessed and happy outcome of doing something that brings pleasure? What if — oh my goodness — reproduction is a reward to encourage people to have a lot of sex? The conventional wisdom is that sex feels so good because it's a reward for engaging in reproductive mating. What if it's the other way around: the possibility of conception encourages people to engage in frequent sex, lovely sex, nature's best remedy to numerous human health issues?

It's all very chicken and eggy, of course. We can't prove either but I can't help wondering whether all organisms, animal and vegetable, derive some benefit from sex (whether it is pleasure, release, or better health) that makes them want to do it again and again. Is it likely that fission "feels" good to amoebas? Errr. You didn't read me saying that. But is it possible? It seems at least as credible as amoebas being driven by a Biblical imperative to multiply.

Which leads me to end this volume and introduce you to the next one, formally known as Volume II of *The Truth About Sex*. I never expected that this book would become a trilogy: I've wanted to write this book for the last fifteen years. My hope in those heady early days was to write a short slim volume covering key points about normalcy and sex. Mainstream publishers, however, were uncomfortable with the ideas — and their unconventional author's notoriety — so, the project kept going back into the hopper, as other projects (including completing my doctorate in Human Sexuality and publishing my last book, *Come Hither*) took precedence. Meanwhile, I kept researching and learning, and adding more and more material to this project in the faith that ultimately it would be published. Still, I dreamed of a slim volume, because, as a reader and a writer, I've become a hard core fan of the short form in the new media-drenched culture.

When I opened my therapy practice in 2000, I began to dig deeper into the heart of sex: its meanings, its patterns, its polymorphousness. Although I started out specializing in kink and fetish sex, these days my practice is a diverse mix of clients, some of whom struggle with common complaints: a loss of interest in sex, problems with orgasm and sexual function, sexual conflicts, relationship issues, body image issues, and other typical questions or concerns that people bring to sex therapists.

Meeting their needs has meant learning enough about basic sex medicine to know when to refer them to medical doctors and to advise them on tests to request and questions to ask — and when to advise them to skip the doctor too. It has meant keeping an eye on new sex studies so I can be up-to-date on innovative theories and treatments. It has meant coming up with original treatment plans, and unconventional approaches that target a person's uniqueness, rather than treating everyone according to a formula. It also has meant keeping up with developments in natural health and wellness so I may recommend effective non-medical approaches to common sex problems. Mostly it has involved an awful lot of thinking about what it all means so that, ultimately, I can help clients find peace with their relationships and sex lives.

And so, for better or worse, I became consumed with the urge to distill what I'd learned into this project, and offer readers the kind of information and advice I've provided to hundreds of clients over the years. Which means this book is bigger than I intended and now, years later, as I sift through thousands of notes and files that have been dutifully copied from desktops to laptops to storage devices for the past decade, the task of sorting through it all and selecting the material to include has been challenging to say the least. To help maintain my sanity, and keep things very organized for readers, I decided the best approach was to do it as a trilogy. Now, instead of one slim volume, I'm writing three slim volumes.

This volume offered the basic grounding in sex theory and history, and addressed the fundamentals of adult sexuality, masturbation and orgasm. Volume II is dedicated to partnered intimacy in all its diverse forms. I'll be focusing my sexological lens on coupled intimacy as it is lived, and poking, prodding and probing the most common penetrative forms of sex (vaginal, anal and oral) on equal footing, as the three most pleasurable penetrative acts adults crave. There's a chapter on swinging, open relationships and polyamory — three rather different types of adult relationships that beg for some clarification, and even a history of marriage that's filled with curious facts.

The second half of the next book explores sexual variations which some adults enjoy as a kind of spicy side-dish to their typical sexual interactions, and which other adults consider the main course itself. Among the variations I explore are sexual role play and the use of fantasy in sex: erotic (i.e., for the purpose of being aroused) gender reversal or transformation; fetish sex; spanking and bondage; and tantric sex.

The final volume will be devoted to sexual health. It may sound like a dry subject but actually this will be the volume that breaks out the real sexual differences between men and women. Split into two halves (male sexual health and female sexual), this volume will answer all the common questions men and women have about their sexual anatomy (size issues, sensitivity, performance), their sexual responses, and sexual impulses they never understood. I provide a state-of-the-art glimpse of the science of sexual health, including preventative tips and advice for all adults, regardless of age, size, or physical challenge. Most importantly, I offer realistic, empowering, and inclusive new models of the normal ranges of male and female sexuality, along with advice for each stage of adult sexuality, from youth to old age.

Finally, although my triad of mini-tomes are not intended as self-help, nor a replacement for working one-on-one with a competent sex therapist, I don't think a sex manual is complete without at least a few tips and techniques. At the end of each book, I offer a series of exercises related to the volume's content. In this case, some exercises you can try to improve your own skills with auto-erotic pleasure and mutual masturbation. They are based on the types of homework I occasionally inflict on clients. If you'd like to sample the Dr. Brame experience, flip there now and try one at home tonight.

May all your orgasms be ecstatic. See you in Volume II.

EXERCISE 1: LOVE YOU IN THE TUB

One of the sadder, stranger phenomena of adult life is that many people are alienated and dissociated from their bodies. As a therapist, I've worked with people who viewed their physical bodies as cages, or as unpleasant weights they were forced to drag around. Some were deeply ashamed about touching their genitals or nipples — and a few were embarrassed that they even had sexual features in the first place.

A great model of sexual health is when you feel that your body (or external self) is as much a part of your identity as mind or soul (your internal self), and when you can achieve a peaceful, integrated balance between body and mind. Lack of body self-acceptance is, in my clinical opinion, one of the chief obstacles preventing adults from pursuing satisfying encounters or achieving satisfaction from sexual encounters.

This exercise is designed to help adults overcome inhibitions about their bodies. Whether the issue is shame at the way your body looks, shame about your genitals, or difficulty feeling safe when you are fully naked, here are two gentle exercises in relaxing your body and mind together.

You should spend a minimum of 30 minutes on this exercise.

Caution: You are allowed to sip a single glass of wine or indulge in any other SOFT stimulant to heighten your senses if you wish. However, these exercises are safest when sober and should NEVER be performed when your judgment is impaired. Any substance which impairs your judgment will also alter your sexual responses, both good and bad.

LOVE YOU IN THE TUB

A warm bath is perhaps the easiest, most relaxing way to begin the process of body acceptance. You can opt for salts or bubbles or even rubber duckies if you like. If you have the means to create a spa experience for yourself (burning a scented candle or incense, dimming the lights) better still.

Armed with your favorite bar of soap, your only task is to wash every part of your body you can reach with slow, gentle movements. Do not speed past any spots that usually make you uneasy. Spend more time with them than usual. Just soap the skin and rub the suds with your fingers from toe to chin. If you encounter an orifice, dip your slippery finger in it to gently cleanse. Separate skin folds, follow contours, take your time. If you find a spot that's interesting, linger there. If you'd like a mantra or words to repeat, try "all places on my body are equal" or "every part of my body is clean."

You can do this with your eyes closed as long as you promise not to swoon under the waterline. While I'm the last person to discourage an orgasm, that's not the point of this exercise. Its purpose is to reacquaint you with every sensual inch of your skin, without prejudice against those parts you usually try to forget or ignore.

If you cannot reach all the parts of your body with your hands, use a gentle bath brush with a soft foam sponge to extend your range. No loofah and no scrubbing please!

LOVE YOU IN BED

Some of my clients dislike soaking in tubs. For them, I suggest they try something similar while in bed.

First, of course, all garments off, so you are completely nude. Next, since lying in bed may not bring the immediate feeling of relaxation that comes from stepping into steamy water, try and create a little calming magic of you own. You may find it helpful to power on your iPod and blow some relaxing music into your ears. Dim the lights, burn an aromatic oil, take a few deep breaths or a sip of wine. Your state of mind is crucial to the experiment, so build yourself a little bubble of contentment before you begin.

I don't want you to soil any expensive sheets with unguents or oils, but please think of this as a full-body massage — only you will be massaging only with the tips of your fingers and not trying to hammer on any pressure points. If you are mechanically inclined, you can think of it as a full body-check to make sure everything is where it should be and feels A-OK. Begin with your toes and slowly work your fingertips over every part of your body you can reach. (If you can't reach some spots, again, use a tool with a soft end to prevent accidental abrasion.)

Although the exercise may arouse you, again, arousal is not its purpose. Focus on really getting to know and "feel" your body — what places feel great? Which ones make you shrivel up inside a little? Do your best not to consciously differentiate your genitals, nipples and anal region from the rest of your body: they are all you and, as the title of this exercise states, this is about loving YOU in your physical totality.

If you enjoy the experience, my advice is to repeat it until it becomes boring. You will experience some benefit right up until that moment because each repetition will give you new insights into the sensual potential of your body and better body confidence overall. If it never becomes boring, and you're brave, ask a lover to try this with you, and see if you can sensually massage each other to gentle bliss.

~ EXERCISE 2: FEEL YOU ~

The follow-up to the first exercise is a more deliberate effort to understand your sexual responses, to become relaxed enough to receive pleasure, and to begin to organize your growing awareness about what really turns you on and what really turns you off.

Most of us walk around in our bodies without ever fully appreciating their incredible capacity for pleasure and sensuality. This exercise operates from the notion that ANYTHING has the potential to feel sexy, depending on an individual's unique chemistry and biology. Most clients who try this exercise come away a bit surprised by how good it felt to tickle or caress a spot they never before considered erotic. You too could be one of those people who never before realized that a certain kind of touch to an arm or thigh would feel almost as good as direct genital contact. This exercise will help you figure that out.

(If you wish, you may chart or journal your responses. Keeping a record of these exercises is most useful to people with significant emotional blocks against nudity and masturbation.)

You can do this in bed or, if you don't have much privacy, behind a locked bathroom door. Again, it's always helpful to inspire yourself with something that relaxes or soothes. It's also fine if you'd like to supplement this exercise with a magazine or erotic toy to get you a little pre-aroused.

This is very much like "love you" but with a focus on erotic pleasure. If you did that first exercise, you are well-acquainted with the full-body self-touch. This time, however, it is not just about fingertips. You are free to pinch, poke, caress, and deliver any other enticing sensation to each part of your body as you go.

It may sound silly on the surface that I'm asking you to lovingly stroke a toe and then to squeeze, slap or tickle it. But until you are sure that your toes don't hold some mystical erotic potential, that is my advice. Treat your entire body as a territory to explore, much as you probably did when you were a little kid (or as you might have if your parents hadn't made you stop). If you wish to try inserting a safe clean object into an orifice, (preferably it will be a sanitized toy designed for the purpose), go right ahead.

CAUTION: *Please sanitize your toy after each insertion into a different orifice. Be careful not to transmit bacteria from anus to vagina or mouth.*

Your goal is to explore all your natural pleasure points. Not just the ones you think should give you pleasure, but every spot that makes you say "ahhh" and "ooooh." Experiment with different sensations. Some clients have used silky or furry fabrics to rev up the sensuality; some try extreme variations and explore intense sensations. That part is up to your personal sexual tastes and sense of adventure.

Finally, don't be afraid of the results. No one but you need ever know that a spot on your neck turns you on like crazy — unless, of course, you wish to share it with a lover and improve your sexual pleasure. Just saying.

You should spend a minimum of 45 minutes to an hour on this exercise.

~ EXERCISE 3: GIVE YOURSELF AN ORGASM ~

An amazing (and amazingly unempowered) fact about women is that many of us depend on other people to give us orgasms, whether it's a boyfriend, girlfriend, or spouse. It is the rare man who doesn't know how to give himself an orgasm but a significant percentage of women remain in the dark about how to achieve a satisfying climax. On the other hand, it's not uncommon for adults of all sexes to feel that masturbation is dirty or wrong, and to avoid it or limit its frequency out of shame.

Thus, this exercise has two separate components: an exercise tailored to women and one tailored to men. It may also serve as a guide for lovers who have not yet mastered the technique of giving their partners orgasms by hand.

ORGASM TIPS FOR WOMEN

If you've never been able to climax from intercourse, relax: over half of all women do not get the clitoral stimulation they need from intercourse alone. Key to female sexual response is a mix of emotional readiness (sometimes called "in the mood" by lay people, and "receptive" by clinicians) and foreplay. Women who can become instantly excited, make love in a flash AND climax are rarer than hen's teeth. For most women, particularly once they hit their late 20s, climax is more elusive and complex.

Assuming you did the first two exercises, you should have a good inventory of how body parts feel and which areas are most sensitive to touch. Using your insights about your body as the template, relax and gently caress any areas you know give you special pleasure (whether or not they are directly sexual). Your goal is to raise your body temperature, warm your vagina with good blood flow, and allow yourself to experience an unthreatening, self-ministered pleasure. Don't rush. Spend at least 10-15 minutes "teasing" yourself with touches to any part of your body that makes you feel sexy.

Experience tells me that most women find their best success with their first solo orgasm by using an adult toy, usually a vibrator. Experience also tells me that each of us should throw away the book (of course, not this one!) when it comes to techniques and expectations. Do not expect success the first time. You're still learning: don't sabotage your success by thinking you can get where you're going the first time you try. Do not expect to hear fireworks — if you hear them, it will likely be after a few experiments, when you've finally mastered your best techniques. Do not drive yourself crazy searching for your G-spot: you may not have one. Even if you do, it may take time to learn how to stimulate it for maximum pleasure. Instead, focus on how you FEEL, not how you think you should feel.

Settle into a fantasy about who you might want to be with right now, or what kinds of sex you would love to be having, or even a beautiful setting for romance. Yes, I'm afraid I have to say it: try to think happy thoughts. In sex, happy thoughts are a woman's best friends.

Begin by gently kneading the mound, gripping softly and then more aggressively. Not all women enjoy the intensity of direct stimulation, so squeezing the front top opening of the vagina (where the lips begin) or exploring between the lips will take you close enough to it to derive some pleasure. Many women, indeed, prefer squeezing or applying pressure against their labia to direct clitoral stimulation. That's why humping (or "outercourse") can bring orgasms: the pressure of the grinding triggers orgasm.

Stroke the labia, inside AND out. Since labia are NOT always sensitive, if teasing and caressing don't feel good, try clamping and slightly pulling them away from the body to see if it helps. While the labia themselves may not bring pleasure, firm manipulations from the outside should create pleasurable sensations on the inside. See if you can get yourself aroused and lubricating just from these external rubbing/groping exercises.

To climax, you will likely need more direct stimulation to the clitoris. Begin to lightly tease your clitoris. If you are not sure where it is, that's okay, I won't make you examine it in a mirror (though I'd be pleased if you felt comfy enough to do so). Just remember it's way in front, just inside the top of the labia, and externally separate from the vaginal canal, just as a penis is externally separate from testicles. You can roll your fingers into a soft fist and gently massage the area or, if you are comfortable, move your fingers around until you find a spot that feels intensely exciting and settle there.

While female orgasm is produced primarily by the clitoris, the vaginal canal is also extremely receptive to fondling and penetration and may (depending on your body) take your pleasure and orgasm to a much higher level. The safest things to insert are your finger and hand; or a clean sex toy specifically designed for penetration. If and when you are great with masturbation, insert the sanitary object of your choice but, for now, keep it SIMPLE please. Learning how to give yourself an orgasm from exotic or otherwise exceptional insertions will be great fun down the road but this exercise is specifically geared to help you reliably give yourself an orgasm the old-fashioned way.

Your entire pelvic region is sex-sensitive — including thighs and behind — so if you find it gets too intense just working on the sex equipment, vary your thrill by moving your hand (or toy) around to other exciting spots. If you get stressed out, stop. Take a break, have a sip of water, slow down. Chances of orgasm are reduced by stress. Try the exercise when you are feeling calmer or more upbeat.

If what you are doing is getting you more and more excited, keep going. If all goes perfectly, at a certain point (different for every woman), you will feel a growing urge for release that propels you into a less-than-fully-conscious state. This is a good thing. Allow the feelings to wash over you. The need to complete the experience will build, as will your focus on what you are doing. Relax into it and let biology take over and do what it is wired to do. The experience of orgasm is subjective but shares some commonalities: you may be more aware of your genitals than any other part of your body; you may feel inarticulate incoherent (normal); your need for release may supplant all other needs. If you can, ride that emotional high, and your body will naturally complete its journey to orgasm.

If you find your desire flagging, your mind racing, and inhibitions popping up, take a break. This is your mind fighting the feeling of vulnerability that comes with surrender to sexual arousal and refusing to give up control. Go back to exercises 1 and 2 for a week and try this again when your body confidence is bolstered by more experience.

If you hit gold first time out, lucky you, but don't make it the standard: accept variability in intensity and duration of orgasms and don't be disappointed if it doesn't happen the same way the next time. Just keep learning about your responses and you will, eventually, figure out how to consistently give yourself wonderful orgasms. Some women are able to climax after just a few moments of foreplay, whereas some women can take half an hour or longer to relax and warm up enough to be ready.

CAUTION: Do not hammer at yourself, with hand or vibrator, when it stops feeling good. Treat discomfort, numbness, pain, and other unwanted sensations as warning signs that your body needs a rest NOW. Stop what you're doing and don't try to fight through pain. Genital pain during masturbation usually indicates an underlying health issue. If anything in this exercise causes pain, you could have a yeast infection, adhesions, or other problem. See your gynecologist to find out what's causing the pain.

Every healthy woman can experience an orgasm. The only secret is not to give up and to understand and accept your body well enough to know that you may need something just a little different to get over the top. This is something to remember through every stage of adult female sexuality, since what you need right now may not be what you needed in the past or what you will need in the future to achieve a soul-satisfying orgasm.

Finally, be aware that small changes in hormones, environment, circumstances, and health can compromise anyone's sexual performance. Be patient and forgiving with yourself and if it doesn't work out today, try again after you've had a good night's sleep. If you're drier than you wish, add a lubricant. You have three options: water-based, oil-based, or silicone-based. According to some recent studies, a lubricant can significantly improve female sensitivity and pleasure. A bottle of lubricant you can rely on will not only improve masturbatory fun but will become a godsend the next time you have penetrative sex with a partner.

ORGASM TIPS FOR MEN

Men usually have very different issues with orgasms from women. Some women do not know where their clitoris is, for example, but I've yet to meet a man who cannot locate his penis. Men are accustomed to handling their penis throughout the course of daily life, whether it's washing it in the shower, using it to empty their bladder, or positioning it subtly for modesty's sake in one's pants. In my experience, the bigger challenge for men is when they switch gears from "penis as tool to urinate" to "penis as aching throbbing organ that needs relief." Overcoming the shame and embarrassment you may feel about masturbation, and the belief that only sex with a partner is "real" adult sex while masturbation is a nasty teenage behavior, is a process that takes a little time and a lot of self-acceptance.

While you can certainly masturbate without the use of lubricants, I generally recommend them to ensure a smooth, slippery, sensual experience. Depending on your penis' sensitivity, whether or not you're circumcised (and even how adeptly you were circumcised), there is always a small possibility that masturbatory rubbing can result in a feeling of soreness. Men may use something as simple as baby oil, though I always prefer water-based products specifically designed for the purpose. They feel better, they work better, and they are the only safe choice when using condoms (which will react poorly with a petroleum-based product).

Most men treat masturbation in a very direct way: they grab themselves and begin to stroke. This is fine if you already feel okay with your penis or, conversely, if you are so uptight you will only allow your penis to feel sexual. Instead of going for the gusto, I often advise men to try and NOT be so goal-oriented about sex — neither with your partners, nor with yourself.

Men (just like women) are loaded with erogenous zones throughout the pelvic region. It's sad to me that so many men just work for an orgasm, rather than a complete erotic experience, so I encourage male clients to work on their sensuality instead. You have potential you probably haven't begun to tap into it. So I recommend that you NOT touch your penis for the first 10-15 minutes of self-stimulation. Focus, instead, on giving yourself the strongest, hardest erection you can by teasing yourself to lust in other ways.

As with fancy sex toys for women, I discourage the use of porn and sex toys UNTIL you know how to give yourself a great orgasm without those assists. You may have developed a rigid behavioral pattern of "needing" porn to get off; it's just a behavior, which means you can (and should) break it. Assuming you're in good sexual health, you should also be able to achieve an orgasm independently, as in nature, without artificial stimulants. That said, once you have mastered masturbatory technique, feel free to look at any images that turn you on. I am NOT anti-porn (heavens forefend), I just know that until you can give yourself orgasms without the bells and whistles, you have not yet given yourself psychological permission to fully savor your own sensual potential.

Not all, but many men also derive pleasure and excitement from their nipples. If you did the first exercises, by now, you should have a clear idea if you are lucky enough to have erotically-sensitive nipples. And, if you do, your foreplay should begin at your chest, with soft, gentle (at first) manipulation of your nipples.

If you do not get pleasure from your nipples (not uncommon among men), there are still lots of lovely spots to stroke and tease. The area between the testicles and the anus is very sensual; the buttocks and anal region are sensitive, as are your thighs and testicles. Begin with light touches, caresses, pinches or squeezes in and around those areas. If it feels strange or awkward at first, close your eyes and imagine a lover touching you in all those places. If you require more intense sensation, increase the pressure or squeeze/slap harder. If you need a goal, make the goal the best erection you can possibly have.

The penis is not as sensitive as a clitoris (there will be in-depth explanations of why and why not in Volume III, but for now I ask you take my word for it), so men doing this exercise don't have to spend quite as much time stimulating other parts (unless you really enjoy doing so, as I hope you will). After about 5-7 minutes, you may be ready for direct stimulation. Put a small glob of lubricant in your palm and you're ready.

Most men will climax from a slow, steady, rhythmic up and down stroking. It can take anywhere from a minute to over half an hour for men to come; don't worry about how long it takes, just focus on how good it feels. If, any point, you feel sore, stop and add more lubricant. Some men hold themselves halfway up the shaft, but I recommend that you try and stroke from the base (where the penis connects to the body) to the head, for maximum stimulation and maximum sexual health too. Muscles in the region will appreciate a full stroke, rather than fast yanks on the upper shaft.

If possible, shift your focus away from "get it over with" and center it on "how much pleasure can this baby give me?" Try different strokes, change up the rhythm of stroking, include lots of interesting sensations (rub or gently caress the sensitive head; use your other hand to play with your testicles or anal region; include any rough touches that you know add spice to your pleasure).

Finally, and most importantly, learn to gain control over your timing. Perhaps the most common male complaint I hear is from men who feel their timing is off, and that they come too soon. Although premature ejaculation can go deeper than a behavioral pattern (early studies suggest it is an inherited trait passed from father to son), in most men, the problem is not biological but psychological. More often than not, they come quickly because they have not developed the skill to delay orgasm. This can be a real detriment in relationships and may make a guy feel insecure or inadequate. Understandably: it is an immature model of male sexual health to assume that a penis is automatically going to do whatever a man wants, when he wants it. A mature and much healthier model is when a man can exert some measure of control (variable though it may be at times) over the timing of his release.

The absolute best way to resolve premature or involuntarily rapid orgasm is not to be contained in a numbing spray or pill: the best way is to train yourself and teach yourself a healthier model of adult male sexuality, i.e., learning how to pace yourself, how to slow down your own excitement, and how (and when) to shift focus so that you don't involuntarily ejaculate before you want to. BE AWARE that sometimes your penis may not cooperate, and you will slip and come faster than you wanted. It can happen to anyone once in a while. But if it happens to you regularly, follow my simple guidelines and, over time, you should be able to considerably improve performance and exert more control over duration.

Here are two guiding principles to help you overcome involuntary release.

1. PENIS AWARENESS

In order to be in control of your orgasm, you have to be aware of your penis — what it is doing, and what sensations it is receiving or expecting to receive. Not just, "OMG, I'm hard," but, "That feels great, what might feel better?" The best orgasms come when you feel comfortable with erotic sensations to your genitals and desirous of making those feelings last.

A small shift of perspective (from "my goal is release" to "my goal is pleasure") can make a world of difference here. As delicious as an orgasm may be, it also signals the end of all the wonderful sensations and emotions we experience during arousal, so why rush? Accept that your penis is not an alien attached to your loins with a mind of its own but rather a sensitive system that is wired to your brain. Being conscious of your penis does not mean being self-conscious; it simply means that the man behind it is aware and in control of his own body.

Longer is better — no, not penis size but the amount of time you can enjoy male sexual foreplay before orgasm. In addition to making you a better sex partner to your lover, for most people the more you delay the orgasm, the more intense the bliss and relief when the moment finally arrives. Premature ejaculations are usually marred by a feeling of disappointment not only because things ended quickly but because you have not built up all the psychological and chemical readiness to allow a complete and healing release. It is healthy and positive to extend arousal until your body is REALLY ready for release. The best orgasms are the result of mind and body united and hungry for bliss.

If you struggle with penis self-acceptance, repeat the LOVE YOU and FEEL YOU exercises until you and your penis are on the same page.

2. STOP. REGROUP. REFRESH

Different schools of thought advise different techniques to help men prolong arousal and delay orgasm. Some therapists favor the "pinch" technique: when you feel yourself nearing orgasm, change the sensation from pleasurable masturbation to an uncomfortable rough pinch on the head of the penis (either side of the urinary canal opening), thus "closing" the hole and waiting until the urge to ejaculate ebbs.

Tantric sex for men devotes a good bit of attention to the values of delayed orgasm, but without pain or discomfort. You can stop for a sip of water or a slice of fruit to re-energize and hydrate. You can move your hands away from your genitals and back to another part of the body that felt good (but not good enough to make you climax). You can take a full break, go to the bathroom, or fix yourself a cup of coffee if you need some caffeinated oomph (no alcohol or drugs, please, because they will distort the experience). Most men simply start thinking non-sexy thoughts to slow themselves down. It works but you run the risk of losing your erection completely if you come up with too many unsexy scenarios out of desperation.

I personally favor the Tantric approach but I never force any one technique on clients because everyone operates just slightly differently. So just follow the basic guidelines (STOP. REGROUP. REFRESH) when you feel yourself about to ejaculate.

These exercises should be repeated routinely until you get expert at delaying your own orgasm. The rewards are pretty fabulous: happier sex partners and, of course, a much happier you.

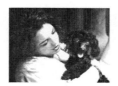

Gloria G. Brame is a sex therapist, bestselling author (*Different Loving, Come Hither*) and poet. She holds an M.A. in English from Columbia University (GSAS 1978) and a Ph.D. from the Institute for Advanced Study of Human Sexuality (2000). Her frequently censored yet astonishingly popular blog, Gloria's Oversexed Mind, covers all aspects of sexual history, and was selected for "Best of SexBlogs 2010" and "NY Sex Bloggers Calendar 2011." Professor of Human Sexuality, Institute for Advanced Study of Human Sexuality (San Francisco); Fellow, Erotic Heritage Museum (Las Vegas); named "Hero of the Sexual Revolution" (Exodus Trust, 2006); regular contributor to The Bilerico Project, the Sexual Health Network, and iFriends Adult Forums. Frequently cited in *Cosmo, Men's Health, Esquire, GQ* and other print and digital media. Google Gloria Brame or follow @DrGloriaBrame on Twitter.